Suspension Calisthenics

For Wolfgang, thank you for designing some of the best suspension equipment on the market.

Table Of Contents

My Journey From Gym Rat To Suspension Fanboy

The book you're now holding is not just about how you can achieve more functional strength and physical control than you ever thought possible.

It's also not just a book on how you can work your muscles as hard as possible while reducing joint stress and improving mobility.

And most of all, this is not just a book on how you can build an ultra space-efficient home gym that costs less than a single dumbbell.

Oh no, my friend, this book is about the two things we humans want more from exercise; total freedom and control over physical fitness. If that sounds good to you, I can't wait to share how you can achieve both objectives with suspension calisthenics.

Who am I?

My name is Matt Schifferle. I didn't grow up using gymnastics rings and suspension straps to strengthen my muscles. The first time I got my hands on a set of gymnastics rings in 6th grade gym class was not a positive experience. I was always a weak and uncoordinated kid.

I eventually fell in love with physical exercise, but I had limited access to exercise equipment. Growing up in Vermont, physical exercise was something you did to help the farmer down the road load in his hay, so good luck finding a suitable squat rack or collection of weight machines. Still, I was a determined kid, so I was always trying to create ways to challenge my muscles.

I started doing basic calisthenics that I learned in Taekwon-Do class, but I didn't understand how to progress the techniques and quickly burned out from doing hundreds of push-ups and crunches daily.

My second attempt at physical training started when I bought some latex strips from the local medical supply store. I had no fancy exercise bands, so I wrapped long Thera-Bands around a post in my basement. That was fun, but the bands would always break, hurting my hands even when I used them while wearing ski gloves.

I never had access to real weights until I attended the University of Vermont. The co-ed weight room was pretty old and antiquated, but I loved using the pec-dec and lat pull-down machine (behind the neck). The downside to the gym was that it was only open for a few hours a week. The limited training hours only reinforced the idea that if I didn't control my access to equipment, then I couldn't have control over my workouts and hence my fitness.

After college, I worked in a shop that sold home exercise equipment and maxed out my credit cards to build my first home gym. At last, I finally had full control over my workouts and ability to exercise. However, I still felt limited by what I could afford and cram into my small apartment. No matter what I purchased, I felt I was missing out on equipment options and the ability to build myself up.

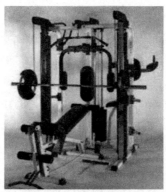

The Prospot weight machine was the central piece in my home gym. I even got rid of my bed and slept on the floor to make room for it.

I loved working out at home but eventually realized that a commercial gym was the only place I could get a real workout. By now, Vermont was finally catching up with modern fitness culture, so there were a few small gyms in my hometown, and I joined one as soon as it opened. I would finally have access to all the equipment I wanted, plus the membership fee was much cheaper than always upgrading my equipment. The only downside was that I became entirely dependent on having access to that gym to exercise. Fortunately, that wasn't an issue as I started working as a personal trainer and virtually lived in the gym, working 16-hour days. I simply figured that becoming entirely dependent on a commercial gym was the only way to build the muscle and strength I wanted.

Around this time, I came across an article in a fitness magazine for a new product called a TRX. It was a very enticing article as the premise was that the device could give you a quality workout with a lightweight and portable piece of equipment.

When it finally arrived, I felt like a kid with a new toy at Christmas. I instantly fell in love with the packaging and design of the trainer. The striking yellow and black appearance and handy carry bag were pure eye candy to me and my desire for strength training autonomy. It's a shame that I thought it was a complete gimmick and quickly left it to collect dust in the corner of the gym.

I didn't even give the TRX a second thought since I was fully on the idea that lifting as much iron as possible was the best way to exercise. Like many young bucks, I had a simple workout plan where I would just put a bunch of weight on a barbell or pin a lot of plates in a weight machine and do my damndest to lift the weight. Form, technique, and range of motion be damned; the only thing that mattered was making more iron move through space. It was a simple plan that worked to some degree, but the good times were not to last.

I loved the long suffer-fests in the weight room, but eventually, my motivation to lift started to wane. Workouts that used to be fun started to feel like a struggle. While I used to attack every set and rep, I now felt slogging through my training as if they were some chore. I also started to experience chronic aches and pains that refused to heal. My knees and hips constantly yelled at me, affecting my sleep.

I was at a turning point in my training career as my body told me things had to change. However, my mental burnout left me little motivation to explore new exercise options. I almost gave up on working out, believing my best days were long behind me. Thankfully, it was then that I came across a book called Convict Conditioning.

The basic idea behind the book is that basic bodyweight drills, like push-ups and squats, can be made easier or harder by adjusting the difficulty of your technique. After reading the book, I decided to challenge myself to a "deload" month where I would do nothing but bodyweight training. Hopefully, I wouldn't lose too much progress as I let my body heal from the heavy lifting.

Much to my delight, I made more progress in my strength training during that month than I had the previous year. I felt my muscles getting stronger, plus I was no longer dealing with chronic pain and stiffness. People at the gym also started to ask me what I was doing as they noticed improvements in my physique. Moreover, my motivation and enthusiasm for strength training came back in full force.

As much as I enjoyed the bare-bones training methods in Convict Conditioning, I couldn't help but feel like there was still room for something else. Something that would take that little world of basic calisthenics exercises and expand it beyond what I was currently doing. Then, I dusted off that old TRX collecting dust in the corner. Now that gimmicky set of straps started to make a lot more sense when I combined it with the basic principles of progressive calisthenics. Suddenly, I was aware of a new world of potential and possibilities to build strength, power, and muscle with little more than just my body weight. Those straps gave me more options and adjustability than just a simple pull-up bar and open floor space. I could replicate almost any weight machine exercise with my body weight. It was also fun to get out of the gym and take the straps to the local playground for an outdoor workout.

The more I used the TRX, the more I imagined ways to improve the design. I've always been a bit of an inventor, and the idea of building my straps became an all-consuming obsession.

Whenever I created a set of straps, I found flaws in my design, so I would go back to the drawing board and design a new set of straps to mitigate those flaws. Over the years, this process has cost me a lot of money and countless hours of experimentation, but it's all been a labor of love. Sometimes, I would start a workout and wind up tinkering around to invent a new set of straps instead.

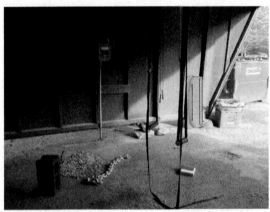

One of my first suspension home gym set-ups cost less than a 45# weight plate on my old Prospot machine but provided a better workout.

Thankfully, modern suspension calisthenics equipment has improved over the years, and many products are much more affordable and better designed than earlier versions. However, I still love to tinker and build my designs, one of which I've included in a later chapter of this book.

It's been over a decade since suspension calisthenics became a cornerstone of my bodyweight training career. I still consider it one of the most enjoyable and rewarding strength training methods I've ever used.

I'm writing this book to share what I've learned and help spread the benefits of suspension calisthenics to you and the world. Gone are the days when effective strength training was a tedious and cumbersome practice that made you dependent on a commercial gym. The dream of an effective workout and the freedom to train anywhere you like is no longer a fantasy. It's well within your reach and far more rewarding than ever.

So without further ado, let's turn the page and dive right into the benefits that can be yours with the ultra-efficient strength training method of suspension calisthenics.

#1

What You Need to Know About Suspension Calisthenics

Suspension calisthenics is a simple and ultra-efficient training method. Some of the most obvious advantages include convenience and portability, but few understand the lesser-known advantages it brings to the table.

Here is a list of some of the most profound benefits of suspension calisthenics.

A wider range of resistance for bodyweight training

Suspension calisthenics is a great tool for filling in the gaps within classic bodyweight exercises like push-ups and pull-ups. I love using suspension straps to train people who are just starting or may be coming off an injury. They bring refreshing flexibility to work around limitations that make conventional bodyweight training prohibitive. I'll also use them to help long-time exercise enthusiasts reach strength levels beyond what they've achieved with classic bodyweight techniques.

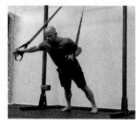 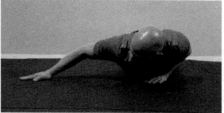

Suspension straps do advanced calisthenics exercises, like archer push-ups, more accessible and easier to adjust than on the floor.

A simple set of suspension straps can transform your menu of training options from a few choice offerings to a plethora of exercises and variations, all within reach of your current capabilities.

Access to accessory exercises via bodyweight training

Effective strength training focuses on fundamental movements like pushing, pulling, and squatting. Basic calisthenics training is fantastic for doing just that, but sometimes it's fun, and even necessary, to branch out into some accessory work like biceps curls or hip abductions.

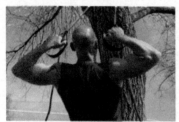 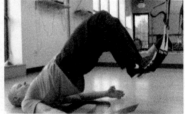

Suspension equipment makes it possible to do exercises like face-pulls or hamstring curls with your body weight instead of relying on a costly machine.

Suspension straps give you access to such accessory exercises without a gym membership or fancy weight machines. It even allows you to practice such exercises and consider them bodyweight training. Now, you can get that sweet pump in your biceps or create stronger hips for kicking with a device you can carry in a backpack!

A portable home gym

Portability and personal freedom go hand-in-hand, making suspension calisthenics ideal for working out on your terms. Plus, getting in a quick workout while on the road can be just the thing to keep the mind and body healthy on lengthy business trips.

Some suspension setups are more portable than others. For example, I only consider gymnastics rings semi-portable due to the size and weight of a basic pair of rings. They are portable, but I usually prefer a basic rope-and-handle setup if I'm traveling light which can easily fit in a coat pocket.

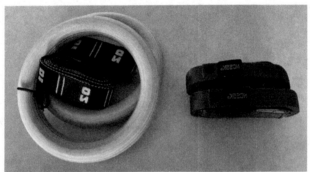

All suspension equipment is relatively portable compared to weight machines or extensive free-weight sets. Some suspension handles are compact enough to fit into a jacket pocket!

I prefer suspension straps to semi-portable options like compact adjustable dumbbells or exercise bands. Suspension equipment tends to be much easier to pack away than a set of hand weights, plus you're still lifting actual weight (your bodyweight) for resistance instead of stretching a rubber band. Bands are a great option, but they rarely offer the level of resistance advanced bodyweight training can provide; plus, you don't have that aggressive resistance curve that comes with using bands. It's the best of both worlds!

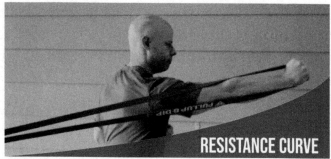

RESISTANCE CURVE

Resistance bands are a viable portable strength-building tool, but they provide most of their resistance when stretched.

A personalized weight machine

Before I learned about suspension straps, I used to be obsessed with weight machine design. I once drove four hours to a shop in Boston to test out a new cable machine. After using it for twenty minutes, I then drove four hours back home. However, it was worth it to get a feel for the equipment.

My obsession faded a bit when I started using suspension straps, largely because I could set them up any way I wanted. Unlike many weight machines that lock you into a supposedly optimal position, you can move freely and place your hands and feet in the best position to work your muscles.

An affordable alternative to a home gym free weights and machines

I once sold a gentleman a pair of 45# weight plates he was adding to his large home gym set up. When I finished ringing up his order, I couldn't help but notice that his two weight plates cost more than both of my home gyms combined. Yes, I had two gyms, one in my basement and one outdoors, for when the weather was nice.

There's nothing wrong, of course, with setting up some free weights for a home gym. However, if you're starting, you can gain a lot of value from a simple set of straps which will likely cost less than a few mismatched dumbbells.

Functional strength

Functional strength is one of those buzzwords misunderstood within our fitness culture. In the early 2000s, the functional fitness craze hit, and suddenly, everyone was giving up heavy squats and pull-ups for stretch bands and Bosu Balls.

The functional fitness idea was born as a reaction to the previous trend to use a lot of fancy high-tech machines and stabilized free weight techniques. In the past, most strength exercises used bodyweight and ground-based free weights. Using such "archaic" methods forced the athlete to stabilize themselves against the forces of gravity. With their reclined benches and controlled motions, the new weight machines decreased the need for such full-body control.

When commercial gyms and strength training became more popular, many people didn't have the athletic skills to use less supportive equipment safely or effectively. It was easier to just sit on a leg press machine and adjust a weight pin than learn how to do a front squat properly. Such machines seemed like a step forward for a while, but time showed that full-body stability was essential for applying your hard-earned strength toward performance on the field or in real life.

Thus, like many trends in fitness, the functional training craze recognized the need for correction but then proceeded to overcompensate with the need for stability and control.

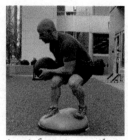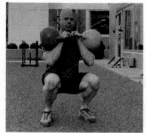

Stability is important for strength training, but compromising stability too much can handicap how hard you can work your muscles.

Bringing back the need for full-body control was a good thing, but placing the body in a very unstable environment can compromise the ability to generate muscle tension. Just think of when you step out onto a patch of ice or try to walk to your seat on an airplane during turbulence. Your environment is so unstable that you become weaker as your nervous system inhibits the neural drive to your muscles to help keep you safe.

The most effective training methods require some total body control and stability, but not so much that it inhibits your ability to contract your muscles powerfully. The most classic and traditional forms of strength training, like basic calisthenics and ground-based free weight exercises, are great examples of achieving this perfect symmetry. Now, suspension calisthenics is the new kid to the party.

Suspension workouts are hardly new, though, as people have used suspension calisthenics for as long as there has been strength training. Athletes have used hanging rings and ropes to achieve this perfect balance between control and strength. Modern-day suspension equipment expands on the discipline and gives you even more options to train every muscle in your body in many ways.

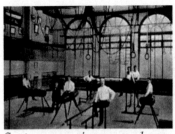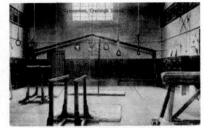

Even the first gymnasiums used ropes and suspension equipment.

Let's explore some of the features and advantages of using such equipment and the different suspension setups you will use.

Suspension setup and adjustment

Like any tool, your safety, comfort, and success with suspension equipment depends on how well you set up and use such tools for optimal training. Even the best equipment will provide a subpar workout if it's not set up correctly.

Here are several tips and considerations I've learned to address to get the most out of your equipment and environment.

Suspension anchoring setup

You can practice suspension calisthenics almost anywhere; however, you need a sturdy anchor point to hang your straps. Finding such a place usually isn't difficult, but different anchor points have advantages and disadvantages.

Suspension calisthenics uses three primary anchoring set-ups. Ideally, your equipment should accommodate all three, but some models may be better suited for just one or two. Here they are with their advantages and disadvantages.

Door anchor points

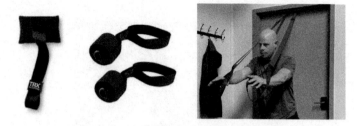

Most suspension setups can be used in a doorway using a pad or bulbous section of a nylon strap that gets wedged between the door frame and the door. Ideally, you place the strap on the inside of the door, so you pull the door against the frame when using the straps. Sometimes this may not be possible, so placing the anchor closer to the hinges is best for support.

It's also incredibly important to ensure that both the door and the door frame are sturdy and do not have any gaps or movement that may release the anchor.

The advantage to using a door anchor is that you can always find a sturdy doorway. This anchor is also ideal for those who travel since most hotels will have a very sturdy door frame that you can use for a workout while on the road.

The downside to working out with the door is that you won't be able to position your body directly under the anchor point. This limitation can hinder your ability to perform some exercises to work against your full body weight. However, you should overcome this limitation by using exercise variations to suit your needs.

Reach height anchor points

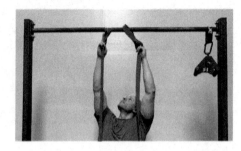

Reach height anchor points are an ideal place to use suspension straps. These usually include a ceiling-mounted anchor point or a pull-up bar that you can reach with a full extension of your arms or standing on your tiptoes.

Having a within-reach anchor point gives you the most versatility and use out of your suspension equipment. You'll be able to adjust your handles to a full vertical and horizontal position. You can bring the handles down to the ground, overhead, and everywhere in between. You can also adjust the width of your anchor points to give you a full range from narrow to a wide setup.

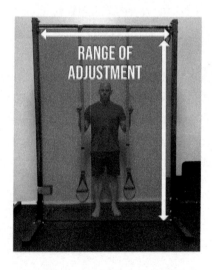

Out-of-reach anchor points

Lastly, you may run into a situation where you have an out-of-reach anchor point. These anchor points allow you to move your body fully underneath your anchor point; however, you anchor the straps to something out of reach, such as a support beam or a high tree branch.

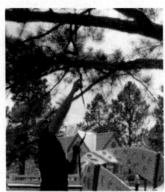

Tree branches are a common example of an out-of-reach anchor point.

The advantage of an out-of-reach anchor point is that it's easy to set up for full extension bodyweight exercises like dead-hang pull-ups and hanging leg raises. Sometimes, these are the only option you may find other than a door anchor while traveling.

The disadvantage to such anchor points is that they often don't allow the handles to go low enough to do a lot of exercises with the foot loops, such as hamstring curls or knee tucks. This anchor point may also not be suitable for some suspension strap designs that require you to reach the anchor point to set up and take down the straps.

Your suspension equipment should accommodate all three anchoring solutions, preferably with as little adjustment or cumbersome accessories as possible. Now let's take a look at some of the ideal designs of the equipment itself.

Single or dual anchor points

The most notable design difference among suspension setups is choosing a duel or single anchor point design. I usually prefer a dual anchor point design since adjusting the handles to any starting width is easier. You can place the anchor points close to each other, giving you the benefit of a narrow base of support and providing extra resistance when pulling handles apart.

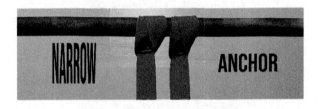

A shoulder-width setup is one of the most stable and is particularly handy for pressing exercises like push-ups and dips. Many people also find this preferable for basic pulling exercises like rowing and pull-ups.

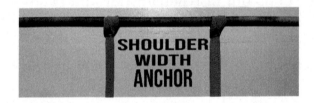

And although it's not commonly used, a wide anchor point solution can be beneficial for providing inward resistance and enhancing exercises like chest flies and hip adductions.

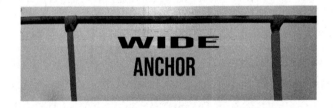

Conversely, a single anchor point setup limits you to a narrow anchor point position for the handles. A narrow anchor is suitable for many exercises but may not be ideal for exercises where you prefer a shoulder-width or wide handle position.

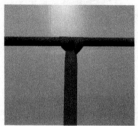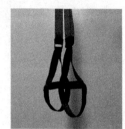

A single anchor point is simple and functional but brings the handles together.

Placing dual anchor points next to each other gives you the same feel as a single anchor point. There are, however, several advantages to consider with single anchor point designs.

The first is that it may provide a simpler equipment design and make building your own suspension equipment easier. Some people prefer a single anchor point design as it's sometimes easier to set up, take down and adjust.

The single anchor point design can often be ideal for out-of-reach anchor points. A dual anchor point design usually requires the anchor points within reach to set up and take down. A single anchor point design is usually attached by throwing one handle over the anchor point for a quick and easy setup.

You can also create a simple clinch knot on within-reach anchor points for a tight and secure anchor.

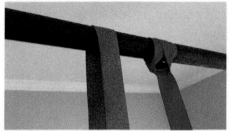

A throw-over anchor (left) is ideal for supports that are out of reach. A clinch anchor (right) holds the support tightly, which offers more stability, but you have to reach it to take down the strap.

I've also figured out a way to overcome the limitations of a single anchor point by hanging a single anchor design with two clinch knots. This anchor can take a little practice and is not as easy to set up and adjust as a dual anchor point design. However, it does at least help you overcome the limitation of a single anchor point, which forces you always to have a narrow handle position.

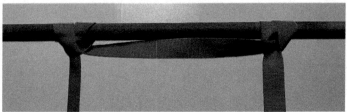

The double clinch knot anchor allows a wider anchor point set up with a single length of strap or rope. Anchor the strap to a single clinch knot, and then throw the other handle over the bar twice (once toward you and once away from you) to create the other knot.

I've even found some suspension designs with a convertible anchor system that can set up both a single and dual anchor point. Such a design can make it the ideal solution for all three anchor point requirements without bulk and attachments.

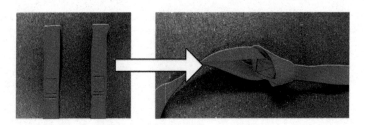

Some dual anchor point designs can be attached to become a single anchor point setup.

Vertical range adjustment

Like with horizontal adjustment, the more vertical range of adjustment you have, the more exercise options and adjustability you'll have in your workouts.

Ideally, you should be able to move the handles to the three most common heights for proper suspension calisthenics training. The first is a full overhead reach for exercises like pull-ups and hanging leg raises. The second is roughly around the waist or hip height for dips and bodyweight rows, and lastly, bringing the handles within a few inches of the floor for push-ups and hamstring curls.

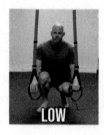 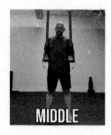 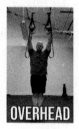

Suspended vs. direct anchor

Technically, a true suspension trainer means that the anchor point hangs from a rope or nylon strap anchored to an anchor point above.

This type of suspended anchor point can be a quick and ideal setup for putting up and taking down your suspension device at a moment's notice. The ever-popular TRX follows just such a design for single and dual anchor point models.

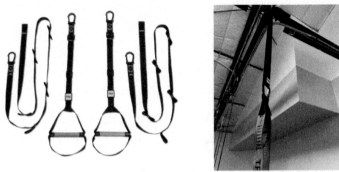

The classic TRX and TRX dual trainers have suspended anchor points that clip onto a hanging strap.

While this design can be novel for quick setup, it can limit your vertical adjustment since you can't bring the handle any higher than the suspended anchor point. It may be much simpler and more practical to anchor the equipment directly to the anchor point and give yourself the option to move the handle with a much broader range of vertical adjustments.

Adjustment buckle and numbered straps

The last thing to consider is the design of the handle height adjustments. Various designs can make it easier or more difficult to quickly change the height of your handles and ensure you have the handles level with one another.

The most common design includes a set of cam buckles that grip the straps tightly when you place weight on them yet release and slide along the straps with the push of a button. You can adjust cam buckles quite easily; however, ensuring your handles are at the same height can be cumbersome.

There are several ways to get around this challenge. One is to use numbered straps to ensure you have each handle at the same corresponding marking.

Another option is to use straps that mount the buckles on the handles. Having the buckles attached to the handles makes it easier to gauge the height and level of the handles since you only have to move the buckles to the height you want. Contrast this with a looping cam buckle design common with gymnastic rings, which may require several attempts to get the handles level and the height you want.

Some single anchor point designs employ a "slipping anchor" where you can slide the straps slightly through the suspended anchor point. A slipping anchor makes it possible to shift your handles to always perfectly level. The downside is that this sliding will compromise your ability to safely shift your weight from one handle to the other since the strap will slip back and forth.

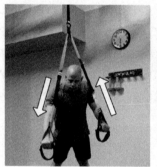 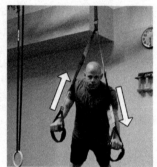

A slipping anchor allows for perfectly level handles but comes at the cost of unilateral stability.

Another clever design is a daisy chain strap where you clip the handles onto set points or D-rings along the straps. This design can seemingly be the perfect solution as you can change the height of the handles very quickly, and you can feel confident that the handles are level with each adjustment.

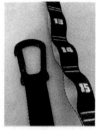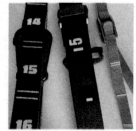

Daisy chain straps and marked suspension straps make adjustment easy.

The downside to this design is that it's only reliable if both straps remain precisely the same length and you anchor them to a level support. Uneven supports, like tree branches or tilting door frames, prevent the handles from becoming level.

Rope or straps

Most commercial suspension designs are constructed out of nylon straps, but some models are made of rope. The primary advantage of rope is that it can save bulk and weight to enhance portability. A rope is also a very handy choice for DIY designs. Nylon strap designs use metal hardware to add weight and bulk, while rope designs use simple knots.

Superfluous accessories

Including many accessories and attachments may seem advantageous, but they can be impractical in daily use. I've seen some suspension designs with so many attachments and accessories that the manufacturer sells a small duffel bag to store and transport it.

I confess that I have gone a little overboard, creating various accessories and attachments for my DIY suspension equipment in the past. At one point, I had close to twenty different accessory attachments for my homemade suspension gym.

Using many accessories isn't necessarily bad, but it adds size and bulk to the design, limiting portability. In addition, having to swap out accessories can add redundancy to your exercise workflow. I'll share some of my favorite designs that incorporate the functionality of door anchors and adjustable handles within a simple design that requires as few add-on accessories as possible.

Twisting handles

Twisting handles are a personal choice, and some people prefer to have handles that twist or solid grip handles that do not rotate like gymnastics rings.

Twisting handles can be particularly handy and more ergonomic for exercises that involve twisting against the hand, like shoulder flies, curls, and triceps extensions. The downside is that rotating handles may feel less stable and can be more challenging to grip during pulling exercises.

Solid non-rotating handles can give you a more stable and secure platform, especially for heavier exercises. The downside is that you'll need to slightly modify your technique and flex or extend the wrist for some exercises.

Foot slings

Lastly, the use of foot slings is another option to consider. Most classic suspension designs have slings incorporated into the handles while using something traditional like gymnastics rings will usually not have them. Foot slings can expand the versatility and functionality of the trainer, but they are not always necessary, and some people prefer to go without them.

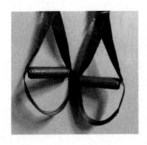 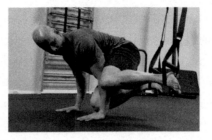

It can be daunting to consider all of these suspension set-up variations. Remember that your ideal suspension setup will mostly depend on your personal preference. I admit that I've become more hyper-focused on such details over the years, but such obsession is not necessary to build a suspension gym from which you'll get great results. So don't overthink it and go with what feels best for you. Your best results don't come from whether or not you use foot slings or gymnastics rings, but how well you use the tools at your disposal, and that's what we're going to dive into in the next section.

Before diving into the meat and potatoes of the exercise portion of this book, I wanted to briefly explain the structure of these sections to guide you for future reference.

These exercises in these six chapters follow my Chain Training theory which I developed several years ago to make programming strength training simpler and easier. Chain Training not only works for basic calisthenics movements but all strength training methods, so feel free to use this approach with any other modalities you enjoy practicing.

The first three chapters are the movement chains, including the push, pull, and squat movement patterns. These exercises use the primary muscles to move the body through space and work to move the limbs relative to the torso. You could consider these three groups the primary tension chains for building your physique and improving overall strength and performance.

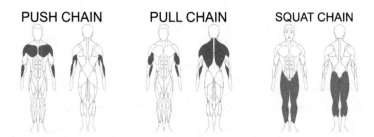

PUSH CHAIN   PULL CHAIN   SQUAT CHAIN

The other three chapters cover your support chains, including the flexion, extension, and lateral chains. These muscle groups are the anatomical chains that run along the length of your body to "glue" the movement chains together. Using these chains is what makes the body move as a cohesive unit and influences your overall physical health.

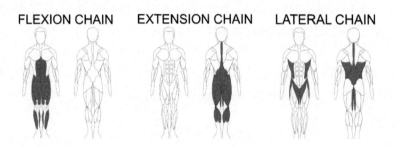

FLEXION CHAIN   EXTENSION CHAIN   LATERAL CHAIN

The world of suspension exercises can be very broad, and some suspension resources list hundreds of exercises you can potentially do with a set of suspension straps. In my experience, most of these exercises are pretty redundant and offer a relatively trivial influence on your health and fitness. Most of the time, these "different exercises" are merely slight variations of one another, and trying to include them can bloat your routine into a time and energy-consuming mess.

That's why I'm going to begin each chapter with only a handful of exercises that are the most potent for conditioning the muscles of that tension chain. Those basic exercises should be more than sufficient to reach your goals. However, the only limit in suspension calisthenics is your imagination, so feel free to modify those exercises however you see fit. You'll still be on the right track if you have the general movement pattern. Each exercise will cover that movement's setup, regressions, and progressions, plus variations to dial in the exercise as you see fit.

Once I cover the basic fundamental exercises for each chain, I will explore some accessory exercises that can help shore up any weak links along that tension chain. Those accessory exercises can be fun, but you probably won't get the best results if you make them the foundation of your workout routine.

So without further adieu, let's start diving into some of the most effective suspension calisthenics exercises for your push chain

#2

Push Chain Exercises

Push chain exercises involve any technique where you push your hands away from your torso against resistance. The muscles involved include the muscles in your chest, shoulders, and triceps, although some lower forearm muscles that open your hand and extend your wrist are also involved.

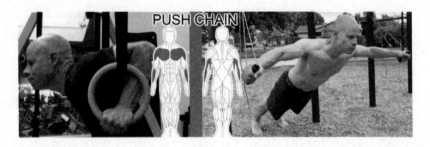

The main compound exercises that deliver the most bang for your buck will focus on various push-up techniques and dips. Let's first explore the most common and fundamental of these exercises with basic push-ups on the suspension straps.

Suspension push-ups

The push-up is one of the most fundamental exercises in all physical training, not to mention the calisthenics universe. Unfortunately, the classic military-style push-up is not suitable for many people, so many struggle to progress with it. In some cases, doing push-ups on the floor can be too difficult for the individual resulting in poor technique to compensate for the lack of strength. The regular push-up is not challenging enough for other people, which leads more advanced athletes to do countless repetitions. Such a practice is fine for building muscular endurance but lacks the intensity to build strength. Performing so many repetitions can also make working out tedious, not to mention time-consuming.

Suspension straps are the perfect push-up companion for several reasons. First, they make it easy to adjust the difficulty of the standard push-to suit your fitness level perfectly. In addition, the ability to move and rotate the handles affords you more freedom to adjust the position of your hands and arms throughout each rep. This freedom of movement helps you unlock a lot of fun push-up variations. It also helps prevent excessive stress in your joints, making for a more comfortable workout. There's a lot to be gained from suspension push-chain work, and here are several key points to keep in mind with the following exercises.

One of the most common mistakes I see people making with suspension push-ups are rubbing their arms against the straps or letting their arms swing out far to the side, placing pressure on the rotator cuffs.

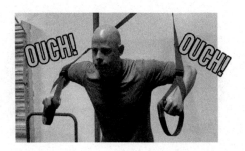

Not only do techniques like this make the exercise uncomfortable and unsatisfying, but they also make it difficult to build the scapular control and stability required to advance towards more challenging push-up variations.

A much more comfortable approach is to start with the straps over the top of the shoulders when your arms are straight. Leave a space roughly half an inch between the strap and your shoulders. As you lower yourself slightly externally, rotate your hands into a neutral position and move the straps alongside your arm as your hands move lower on your torso. It may help to think of moving your body slightly forward of your hands as you lower yourself down. It's OK if your arms gently touch the straps, but there shouldn't be any pressure on the straps against your arm to irritate or chafe your skin.

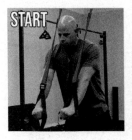
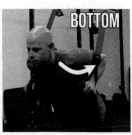
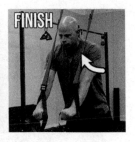

From there, push yourself back up by driving your hands forward and slightly upward to move the straps along your arms and shoulders. Be sure not to "wing out" your elbows so you don't press your arms against the straps while pressing up.

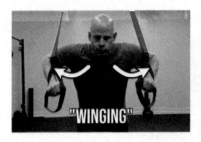
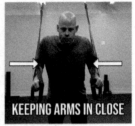

"WINGING" — KEEPING ARMS IN CLOSE

Performing push-ups with this variation will undoubtedly be more challenging, but it's also more effective. Don't be afraid to use lower levels of progression in your technique.

Another tendency with strap push-ups is to let the hips sag while doing the exercise. Suspension push-ups require more shoulder and core stability than traditional push-ups on the floor or a stable surface. You may find your push chain has plenty of strength to perform the exercise, but it may take a bit of practice to ensure you have the core stability to maintain full-body control.

"Pigeoning" or drooping the head is a common mistake when doing push-ups, which can place stress on the neck and compromise stability. It's easy to do as we all receive a lot of environmental feedback through our eyes. Reaching the eyes closer to the floors can make it seem like you're moving lower than you are.

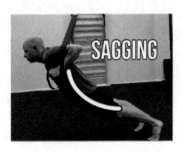
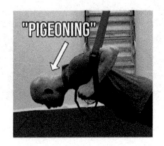

SAGGING — "PIGEONING"

The simplest way to overcome these tendencies is to focus on bringing your chest closer to the floor instead of your eyes. Moving your chest closer to the ground will help you avoid reaching forward with your neck, but it can also help you keep a straighter body position.

You may have heard various opinions on what position you should keep your shoulders in while doing push-ups. Some experts claim it's best to keep your shoulders down and back, while others may recommend pushing the shoulders forward. Both perspectives are valid, but the best thing to do is allow your shoulder blades to move, at least a little, to allow an easier and more natural motion.

It can take some practice, but you'll find that the most natural motion is to push the shoulders forward and even slightly upward toward your ears at the top of each rep. Pull your shoulder blades back and down away from your ears as you descend to "pack" your shoulders. This motion should be easier to manage if you pull your arms close to your sides while bringing the straps along your side.

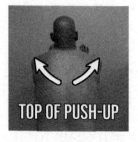 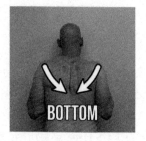

Above all, this scapular motion should help you avoid the dreaded "push-up hunch," which can rob your muscles of the tension they need to grow big and strong while also adding stress to your joints.

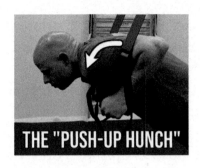

THE "PUSH-UP HUNCH"

Like all basic calisthenics techniques, the push-up is an exercise you can always improve upon and master over the length of your training career. No one ever fully masters it, just as an artist never paints the perfect picture; there is always more to learn and improve upon with the basics. So the key points above are certainly not a comprehensive list of how to perfect the push-up. They are more like a good starting point upon which you can build.

First Level Push-Chain Exercises

The first level push chain exercises place great resistance along your chest, shoulders, and triceps muscles. These are the most fundamental pushing exercises in strength training and are responsible for most of your pressing strength and muscle development.

While most exercises within a tension chain work the muscles the same way, the push chain differs depending on the angle you use. While there is some difference in muscle activation, you should still do your best to use your entire push chain for these exercises to ensure you're working everything. Still engage your triceps and chest with overhead work, even though some might classify that as a "shoulder" exercise. This approach will help you work more muscle, but it will also provide more stability in your shoulders and decrease the risk of injury.

These exercises are also second-level back exercises. You'll want to keep some tension in your back to provide scapular stability. This advice especially applies to dips.

Lastly, I encourage you to play around with hand positions and the width of your hands for these techniques. You can explore fun and challenging variations of most exercises by changing your upper body support base.

INCLINE TO PRONE PUSH-UPS

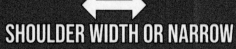

ABOUT 6" ABOVE THE FLOOR

SHOULDER WIDTH OR NARROW

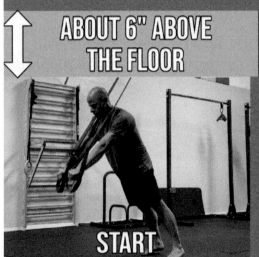

START

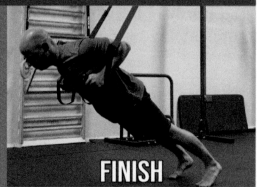

FINISH

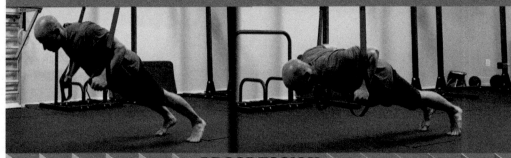

PROGRESSION

NOTES:

Incline push-ups are the best place to start if you're new to suspension push-ups. Be sure to keep your core and glutes tense to avoid sagging as you descend, and focus on pulling your shoulders down and back as you lower your lower chest between your hands.

Progress by moving your feet back to place more weight on your hands. Feel free to rotate your hands as you wish to make it easier to keep your arms tuched in to your sides.

R.T.O. PUSH-UPS

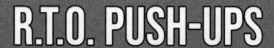

ABOUT 6" ABOVE THE FLOOR

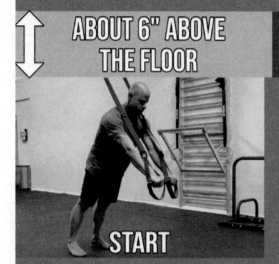

START

SHOULDER WIDTH OR NARROW

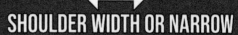

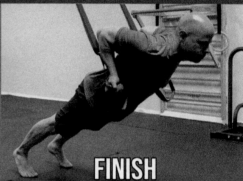

FINISH

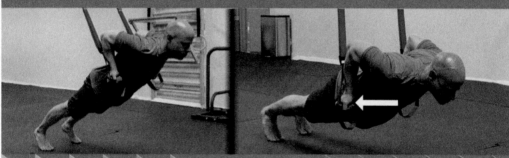

PROGRESSION

NOTES:

RTO (Rings Turned Out) push-ups are a challenging push-up variation that brings a lot of tension into the chest and helps to "pack" the shoulders down and back. Be sure you achieve a full rotation of the hand so your knuckles face forward at the top, and back at the bottom. Try touching the handles to your side at the bottom of each rep.

You can progress two ways. 1) Backing yourself up just as with normal push-ups and 2) reaching your hands back closer to your hips at the bottom of each rep.

ARCHER PUSH-UPS

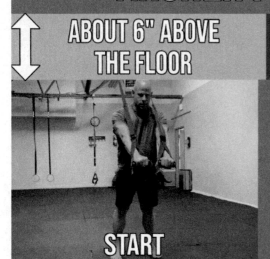

ABOUT 6" ABOVE THE FLOOR

SHOULDER WIDTH OR NARROW

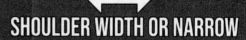

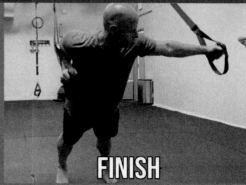

START

FINISH

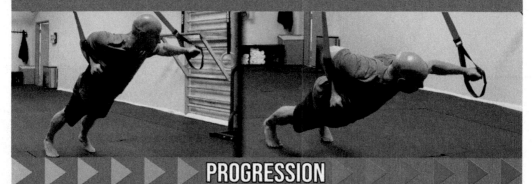

PROGRESSION

NOTES:

Archer push-ups are a great introduction to unilateral push chain training. The goal is to load most of your weight on the pressing arm while the outstretched arm assists against rotation. Don't make the mistake of still keeping your weight 50/50 between each arms as if you're doing a press and fly combination.

Progression is accomplished by backing up to place more weight on your hands. You can also be mindful of how much weight you're loading on your pressing arm and "leaning" more on your pressing arm.

SINGLE-ARM PUSH-UPS

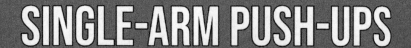

ABOUT 6" ABOVE THE FLOOR

SINGLE STRAP ANCHOR

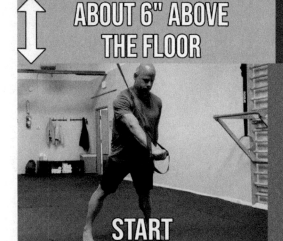

START

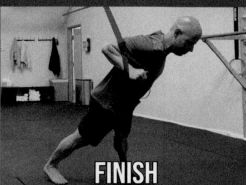

FINISH

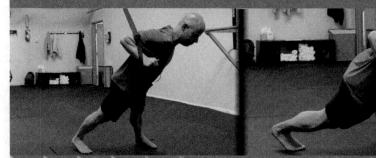

PROGRESSION

NOTES:

Single-arm suspension push-ups are a real challenge! The strap of the trainer wraps around the side of the body and places considerable torque on your torso, so you'll use a wide stance and allow the body to twist toward the pressing arm.

Progression follows the same strategy as other push-up variations where walking back places more weight on the pressing arm. You may need to twist more the lower you go.

FOOT-SUSPENDED PUSH-UPS

ABOUT 10" ABOVE THE FLOOR

NARROW OR SHOULDER WIDTH

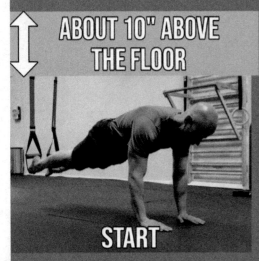
START

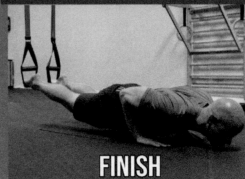
FINISH

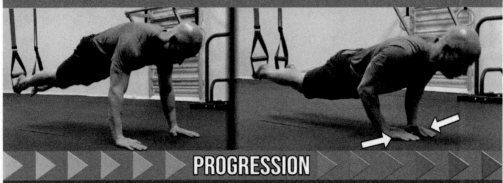
PROGRESSION

NOTES:

Foot-suspended push-ups open the potential for normal floor-based push-up progressions while slightly loading more weight on the hands due to the elevated feet. They also place more resistance on your abs to keep your body tight, so be sure to tense your core and glutes extra hard.

Progress this technique with placing your hands closer together over time. Doing so will not only be more challenging, but will condition the joints for further progressions.

SHIFTING PUSH-UPS

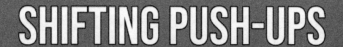

↕ ABOUT 10" ABOVE THE FLOOR

↔ NARROW OR SHOULDER WIDTH

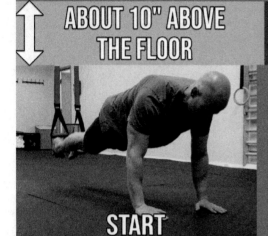

START

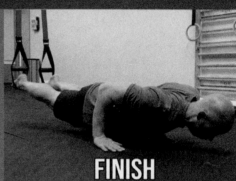

FINISH

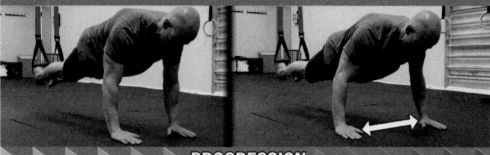

▶▶▶▶▶ **PROGRESSION** ◀◀◀◀◀

NOTES:

Shifting push-ups are an advanced foot-suspended unilateral push-up variation. Start in a normal push-up position, and descend between your hands as like a normal push-up. At the bottom, shift your weight to one side pulling your chest over one hand. Continue to shift over the other hand before returning back to center and pushing yourself back up.

Progress by placing your hands wider apart, so you shift more weight from one side to the other. You can also shift further over your so your hand is more under you.

ARCHER PUSH-UPS

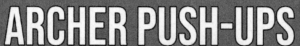

ABOUT 10" ABOVE THE FLOOR

NARROW OR SHOULDER WIDTH

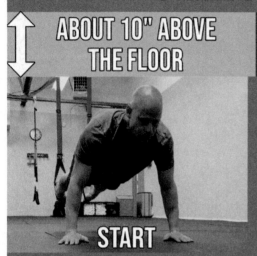

START

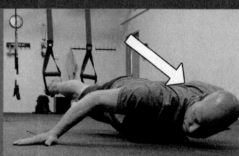

FINISH

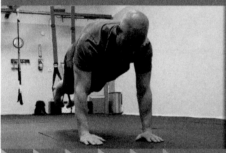

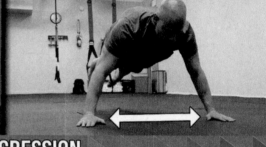

PROGRESSION

NOTES:

Archer push-ups are similar to shifting push-ups, but you immediately shift your weight onto one arm as you descend. This places much more resistance on the pressing arm throughout each repetition. You can complete all reps on one side at a time, or alternate.

Progression is achieved by placing your hands further apart so you place more weight onto the pressing arm, and less weight on the assistance arm.

SINGLE ARM PUSH-UPS

↕ ABOUT 10" ABOVE THE FLOOR

↔ SHOULDER WIDTH OR WIDE

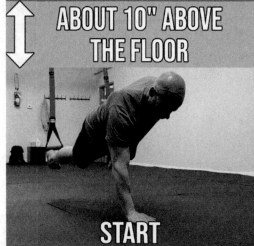

START

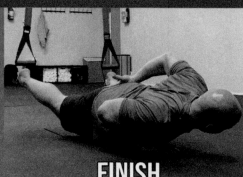

FINISH

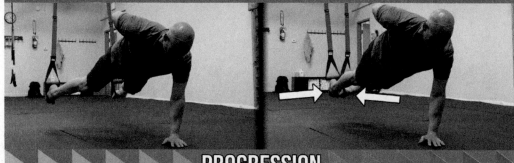

▶ ▶ ▶ ▶ ▶ **PROGRESSION** ▶ ▶ ▶ ▶

NOTES:

The foot-suspended single-arm push-up is one of the most challenging push chain exercises in existence. You'll want a wide anchor point for stability but be sure to keep your lats super tense to also stabilize should shoulder. You may also wish to twit your torso a bit to compensate for rotation.

If you're crazy enough to seek out some progression, try bringing your feet closer together so you have to provide more stability with your pressing arm.

DIPS

AROUND HIP HEIGHT

SHOULDER WIDTH OR WIDE

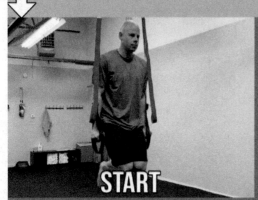

START

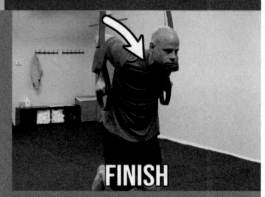

FINISH

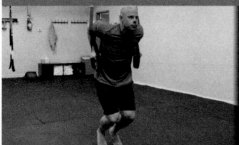

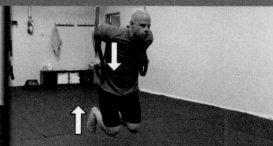

PROGRESSION

NOTES:

Strap or ring dips are more challenging than doing them on stable bars, but they can also be more rewarding. The trick is to keep your back engaged to pull your shoulders down and back for stability. Keep your ams in close and move your torso slightly forward as you lower down.

You can start by using your legs to assist off the ground and reduce lower body assistance over time. You can also progress by descending lower.

SHOULDER PRESS

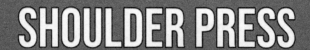

ABOUT 10" ABOVE THE FLOOR

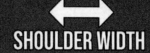

SHOULDER WIDTH

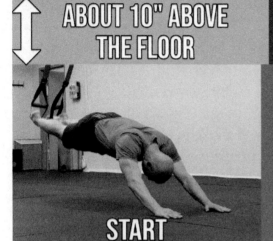

START

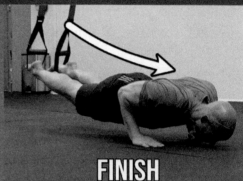

FINISH

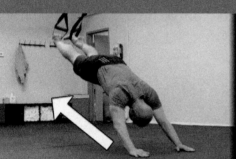

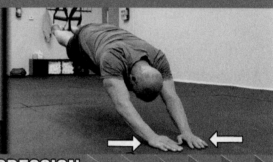

PROGRESSION

NOTES:

This shoulder press variation offers a big range of motion in the shoulders. Place your feet in the straps and walk yourself back 3-4 feet. Stretch out and drive your head between your arms. Lower yourself down and forward of your hands. DON'T GO TO FAILURE! You want to save energy in your arms to safely walk yourself back down.

You can progress two ways. 1) Walk back further to place more weight on your hands and 2) bring your hands in closer to one another.

Second level Push-Chain Exercises

These exercises are some of the best bodyweight techniques for bringing some focused tension into the chest, triceps, or shoulders. While these may be classified as "isolation" exercises, I encourage you to still use as many push chain muscles as possible in each exercise. Remember; don't isolate, *integrate!*

There are many variations of each of these exercises so play around with changing your hand positions, or even integrating various tools to change things up. Loop some hand towels in your foot slings to make the triceps press feel like you're using a triceps rope. Try putting a slight pulse in the bottom of the chest fly to really fry your pectorals. Or you can place your hands wider apart or closer together during the Y-fly to change how the exercise feels on your shoulders. Be creative!

Lastly, these techniques are meant to supplement your first level push chain exercises. These exercises can feel very satisfying, but they shouldn't become the primary focus of your workouts. Think of them as accessory or add-on techniques that you spend about 20% of your workout doing. You'll get the most value from the bigger compound exercises I covered earlier.

TRICEPS PRESS

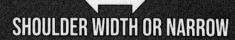

AROUND HIP HEIGHT

SHOULDER WIDTH OR NARROW

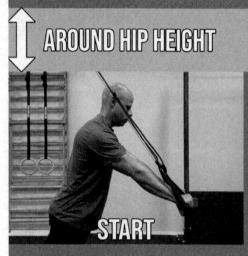

START

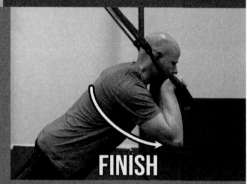

FINISH

PROGRESSION

NOTES:

The triceps press is a very intense upper arm exercise that focuses on using the triceps for elbow extension while keeping the back locked and stable. The key is to lower yourself down by driving your elbows forward under your hands. Your arms shouldn't lift up so you should lower your chain between your hands.

Progression is simple; just step back to place more weight on your hands.

CHEST FLY

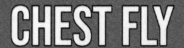

6" OFF THE FLOOR

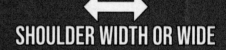

SHOULDER WIDTH OR WIDE

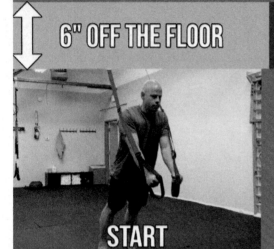

START

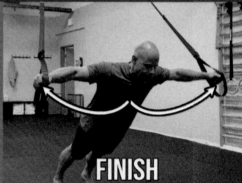

FINISH

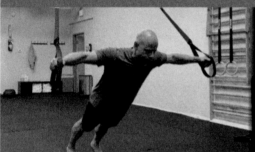

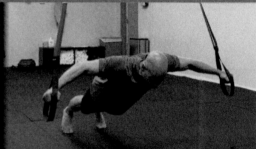

PROGRESSION

NOTES:

Chest flys are a great finisher move for the chest right after a push-up workout. Start with your arms straight and your hands in front of your lower chest. It's okay for the straps to wrap around your shoulders. Keep your body tight as you open your arms to lower yourself down. Pinch your shoulders together at the bottom.

Progress by stepping back to place more weight on your hands.

Y-FLY

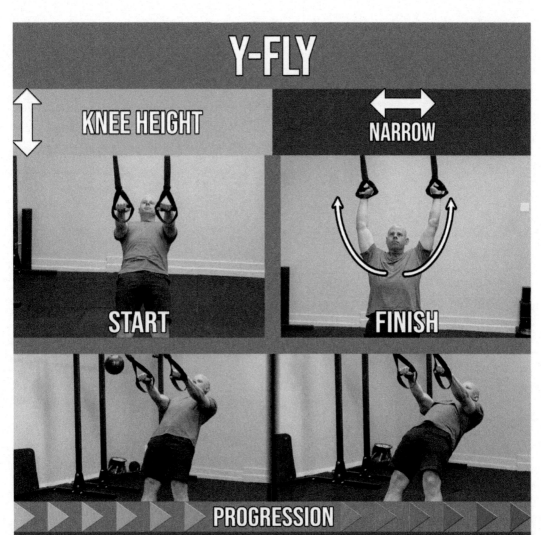

KNEE HEIGHT

NARROW

START

FINISH

PROGRESSION

NOTES:

Y-flys are a shoulder isolation exercise similar to doing a dumbbell lateral or front raise, but with additional benefits for the traps and rotator cuff muscles. Start by facing the anchor point and lean back with your body slightly arched. Pull your arms up and slightly outward while keeping your arms straight. Keep your glutes and hamstrings tight and elevate your shoulders as you lift.

You can progress by stepping forward, but you won't need to take a big step. Even moving forward a few inches can make this exercise very challenging.

#3

Pull Chain Exercises

Suspension pull chain exercises are some of the most effective tools for building up your entire back, biceps, and forearm muscles. These techniques are also a great supplemental way to maintain the muscles that run along your spine and support your lower back.

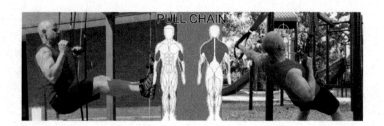

Suspension back exercises offer two big advantages over similar exercises with freeweights and weight machines. The first is the reduction of stress on the spine and lower back. You don't need to hinge at the hips or bend over to perform rows as you would with bent-over rows. The second is suspension pulling exercise requires total body control from head to heels. This total body control helps you work your body as a complete functional unit, as compared to a weight machine.

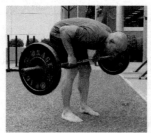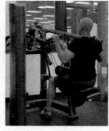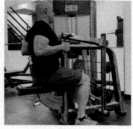

Free weight and machine back training can some with some downsides.

Using suspension straps gave me the best of both worlds. Performing exercises like rows, biceps curls, and rear flys allowed us to work our pulling muscles as hard as we could stand with almost zero shearing stress on the spine and lower back. Furthermore, we still needed to use our lower body to stabilize our body position.

Another suspension advantage is the freedom to change handle placement and rotation. You don't need to bother with clutter-inducing accessories to place your hands at various widths and angles. Suspension handles can accommodate all of those positions and more.

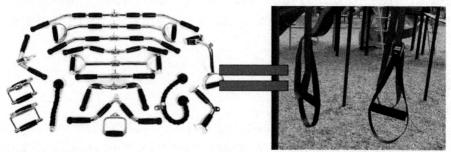

A simple set of suspension straps can replicate almost any weight machine accessory handle giving you endless workout variations.

These various grips are great for changing the "flavor" of your exercises, but they can also be cumbersome and limiting. I usually found myself frustrated with such dedicated grips as they were never quite the right fit.

Suspension handles are the ultimate solution since you can palace them at any height, width, and angle. You can even rotate the handles as you pull if you wish, which can help minimize elbows strain.

A simple set of suspension straps may be the ultimate tool for developing your pull chain safely and ergonomically. The techniques are pretty simple; you just grab hold and pull; it's as simple as that. There are a few things to keep in mind regarding suspension pull-chain training.

Rotating handles can be harder on the grip

Rotating handles can be more challenging to hold on to, especially for heavier pulling exercises like pull-ups and single-arm rows. For this reason, many prefer to use gymnastics rings to afford a stronger and more stable grip.

I prefer a rotating handle to challenge my forearm muscles and build a stronger grip. It can take some time for your grip muscles to get strong enough to handle the heavier training, but I just look at is an effective way to shore up a potentially weak link in the pull chain.

Elbows up or in tight?

It's not so much a mistake, but one of the most common hang-ups I find athletes make with pull chain exercises is to use their arms at around a 45-degree angle. Such a technique isn't a bad thing, but it's a middle ground between tucking your arms in or pointing your elbows to the side. It's fine to use but doesn't pack the same punch as either position.

I recommend keeping your arms close to the body or straight out, like with high rows and rear deltoid flys. Suspension straps make it easier to achieve and maintain these two arm positions. I recommend adhering to those positions as closely as possible when doing pull-chain work.

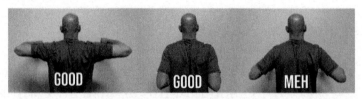

Maintain full-body extension and pack your shoulders

Hunching up the shoulders is another common issue that can compromise your training effectiveness and increase stress in your joints. These issues can be especially prevalent during exercises that place your body in a more upright posture, like curls and pull-downs.

Keeping your entire backside tight, especially your spinal erectors, glutes, and hamstrings, can slightly extend your body. Doing so will help pack your shoulders down and back to ensure you have tension on your back and biceps. It's also a good way to prevent your weight from shifting to your toes to maintain resistance at the top of more upright exercises.

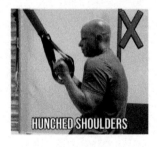
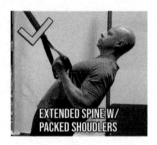

These are just some basic principles to keep in mind but always listen to your body. These guidelines should help reduce stress in your joints and increase the tension in your muscles, but always make any modifications you see fit to make the exercise work best for you.

First level pull chain exercises

Basic pull chain exercises come in two flavors; vertical and horizontal. While rowing and pull-ups are usually considered two very different exercises, I encourage you to blur the lines between those two distinctions.

These pulling exercises use the same muscles to produce the same motions at the same joints. You have shoulder extension coupled with elbow flexion along with isometric grip work in all of these exercises. Theoretically, there shouldn't be much difference in how each of these movements feels aside from how hard the muscles are working. So take the time to contemplate why one pulling exercise might be really hitting your lats while another might leave your lats feeling like they are hardly working at all. Most of the time, the difference is due to a lack of muscle activation than anything specific to the exercise itself.

ROWS

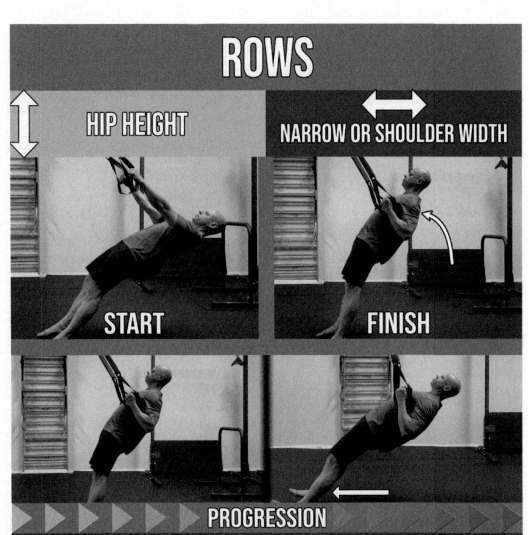

HIP HEIGHT

NARROW OR SHOULDER WIDTH

START

FINISH

PROGRESSION

NOTES:

Bodyweight rows are a pull chain staple. Doing them is simple, just lean back and pull yourself up! Make sure to keep your body stiff so you don't "buck" with your hips. Also, keep your wrists straight at the top of each row. Pull your arms in tight, or out to the side to emphasize the upper back.

Progression is accomplished by stepping forward to angle the body down and place more weight on your hands. You can also progress by moving your feet closer together; creating a narrower base of support.

ARCHER ROWS

HIP HEIGHT

NARROW OR SHOULDER WIDTH

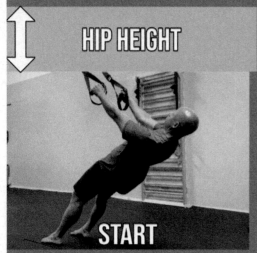

START

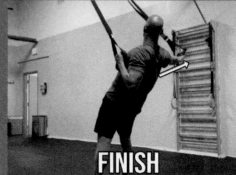

FINISH

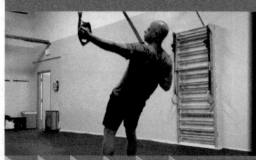

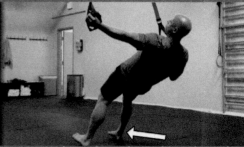

PROGRESSION

NOTES:

Archer rows are a dynamic way to start doing unilateral pull chain exercises. These are just like regular rows, but you extend one arm out to the side while placing most of your weight on the other arm that pulls you upward. Be ultra careful not to hunch the shoulder of your rowing arm to thoroughly work your back and biceps.

Progress this technique the same way as your rows, by moving forward. Using a more narrow stance can also make this a very challenging technique.

SINGLE-ARM ROWS

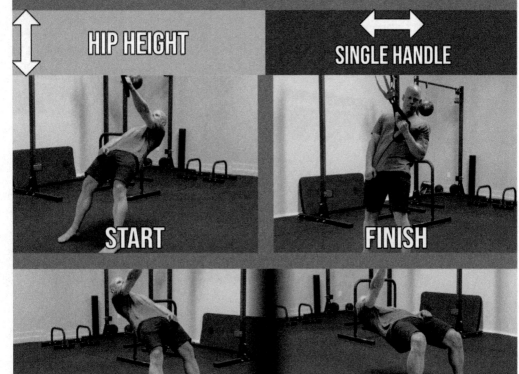

HIP HEIGHT

SINGLE HANDLE

START

FINISH

PROGRESSION

NOTES:

Single-arm suspension rows are similar to bodybuilding dumbbell rows, but with far more challenge throughout the full body. Your entire backside needs to work hard to stabilize your body, especially your glutes and hamstrings. Be sure to push extra hard into the heel of the opposite leg.

Progression happens several ways. 1) You can walk forward as with other rows. 2) Bring your feet closer together. 3) Straighten your legs out as these are usually done with your knees bent at a ninety degree angle.

SEATED PULL-UPS

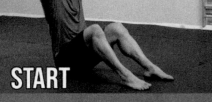

↕ ABOUT WAIST HEIGHT

↔ SHOULDER WIDTH

START

FINISH

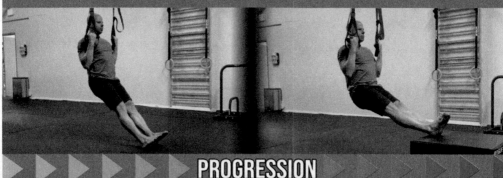

▶ ▶ ▶ ▶ ▶ ▶ PROGRESSION

NOTES:

Seated pull-ups are the ideal way to begin vertical pull chain training. They place less weight on your hands by keeping your feet on the floor or an elevated surface. This position also makes it easier to keep the shoulders "packed" down and back. Just make sure not to push too hard into your feet causing your hips to lift up turning the exercise into a row.

Progress by straightening your legs or place them on an elevated surface.

FULL B.W. PULL-UPS

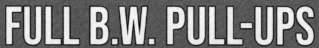

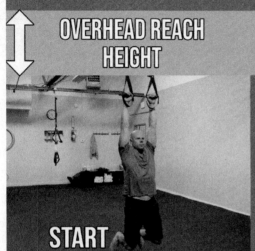

OVERHEAD REACH HEIGHT

START

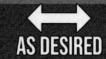

AS DESIRED

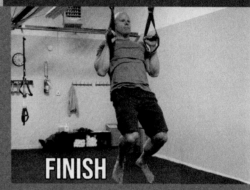

FINISH

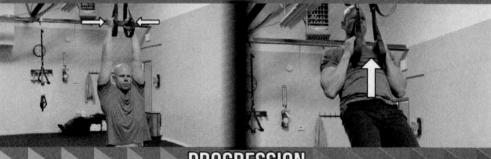

PROGRESSION

NOTES:

These are the classic pull-up technique which makes you work with your full bodyweight. These are less stable than doing them on a solid bar, so be ready to feel your back and arms working harder. Keeping your feet apart can help with this instability. Do your best to maximize your range by fully straightening your arms at the bottom and pulling your chest to your hands at the top.

You can use any hand width you like, but progression is done by moving your hands closer to prepare for more advanced pull-ups.

ARCHER PULL-UPS

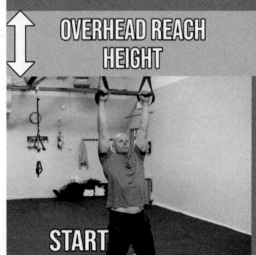

OVERHEAD REACH HEIGHT — START

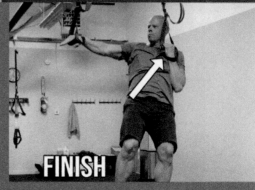

WIDE — FINISH

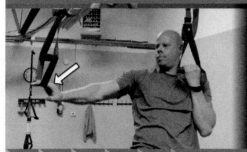

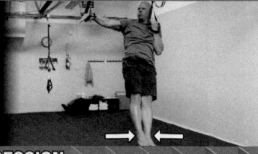

PROGRESSION

NOTES:

Like archer rows, archer pull-ups shift more of your weight to one arm as you lift yourself up. Start with a standard bottom pull-up position and pull yourself up and to one side. Return to the middle and repeat for reps before doing the same on the other side.

Use a wide anchor point set up, and go wider to progress. You can also place more weight on your pulling arm by placing your assistance arm on the foot sling. Keeping your legs together can also make this more challenging.

SINGLE-ARM PULL-UPS

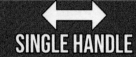

OVERHEAD REACH HEIGHT

SINGLE HANDLE

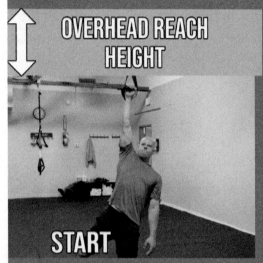

START

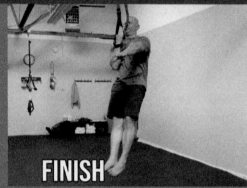

FINISH

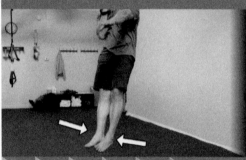

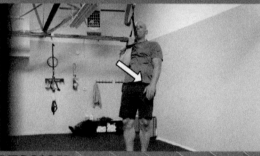

PROGRESSION

NOTES:

Single arm pull-ups are supremely difficult, and doing them suspended only ups the ante by making them less stable. Add in a rotating grip and these are in a class all by themselves.

Progression is all about making the technique as strict as possible. Keeping the legs together, and opposite arm down can really make this an ultra difficult exercise.

Second level pull chain exercises

As with the push chain, these second-level exercises break up the pull chain and emphasize various muscles by primarily moving at a single joint. Do your best to integrate as many muscles as you can with each exercise to provide stability and control. This rule especially applies to keeping your hamstrings and hips tense while leaning back during rear flys and biceps curls.

Some of these techniques are a lot of fun when you use towels including the biceps curls and rear deltoid fly. As always, there are many variations to each of these exercises, so this is far from a comprehensive list. Refer to the pull chain video playlist on the Red Delta Project YouTube channel for more variations.

FRONT LEVER

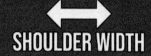

HIP HEIGHT OR AS PREFERRED

SHOULDER WIDTH

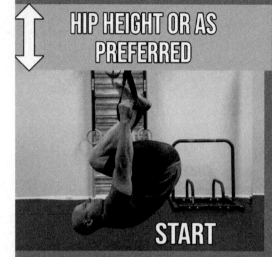

START

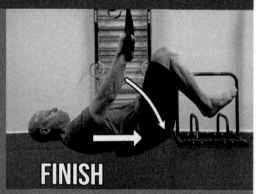

FINISH

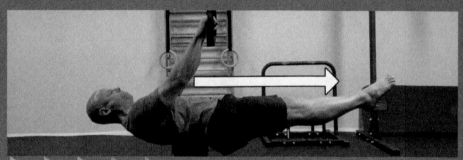

PROGRESSION

NOTES:

A classic "skill" exercise in calisthenics, the front lever is a very intense shoulder extension isometric exercise. It works the entire back, but mostly relies on working at one joint which is why I consider it a second-level move.

Progression is achieved by extending the body. This is done through reaching out with the legs, but don't forget to also extend your spine as well so you don't stay hunched up.

BICEPS CURL

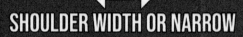

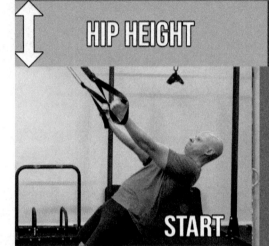

START

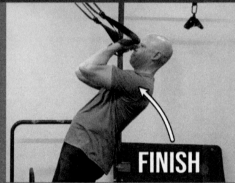

FINISH

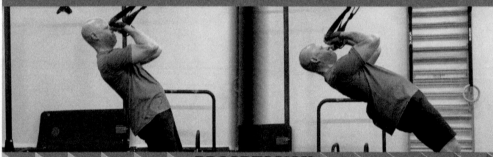

PROGRESSION

NOTES:

The basic suspension curl is a great way to target the biceps, but you still want to keep your full back engaged to maintain a strict technique. Be sure not push your elbows upward slightly to prevent pulling them to your sides which makes the exercise a row. Aim to pull your hands to your face somewhere around your cheek bones.

Progression is achieved by moving forward to place more weight on your hands.

REAR FLY

ABOUT KNEE HEIGHT

NARROW

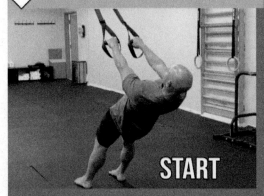

START

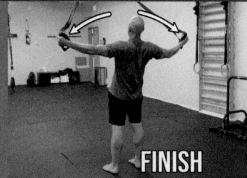

FINISH

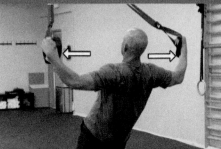

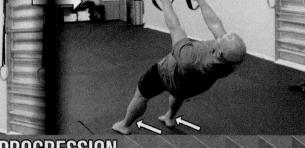

PROGRESSION

NOTES:

Rear "delt" flys are one of the best ways to target your upper back and shoulders.
Beware of the tendency to bend your arms while pulling your hands apart.
Bending the elbows isn't dangerous, but if does reduce the resistance of the exercise.
Keep your weight on your heel to avoid losing resistance at the top of each rep.

you can progress two ways; either by making your arms straighter, or by walking your
feet forward. You won't need to move them forward much, a few inches will do just fine.

LAT. PULL-DOWN

ABOUT KNEE HEIGHT

NARROW

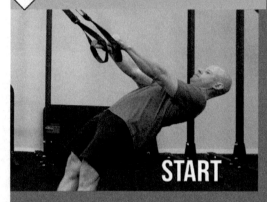

START

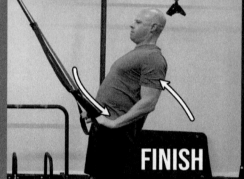

FINISH

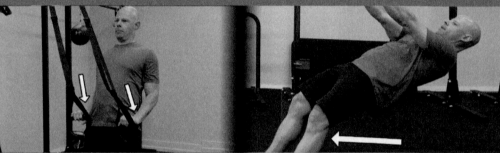

PROGRESSION

NOTES:

Suspension lat. pull-downs are sort of like dynamic front levers. You're pulling yourself up by almost exclusively extending your shoulders. You could think of this move as a very low row as you pull you hands down toward your hips. Bend your arms slightly as you pull so you maintain resistance on your hands, while also pulling your elbows back behind you. Keep your body slightly extended to keep weight on your heels at the top of each rep.

You can progress this move by moving forward, or trying to push your hands lower at the end of each rep.

#4

Squat Chain Exercises

If there's one muscle group that gains a massive benefit from suspension calisthenics, it's the squat chain. However, even die-hard bodyweight enthusiasts have lamented that calisthenics can be great for the upper body. Still, the discipline falls short when training the lower body.

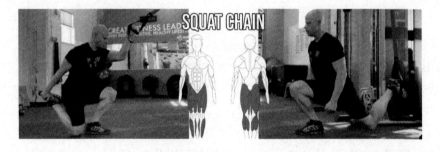

Those well versed in the world of progressive calisthenics understand there's a lot of potential to develop the legs with bodyweight training. Unfortunately, few people explore such potential as advanced squat-chain calisthenics remains out of reach of many athletes.

It's no secret that modern living has most of us sitting down. While excessive sitting can have a negative influence on your lower body strength. How sitting impacts your stability and mobility is the true threat to your leg strength.

Sitting requires a fraction of the lower body mobility used to perform a deep range of motion squat. Furthermore, the supportive design of a chair means we need almost no stability throughout our hips to hold ourselves in place. The result is that most of us have very handicapped hip stability and mobility levels. These inadequacies impede your lower body performance and ability to strengthen your legs with progressive bodyweight training adequately. It's no wonder that many will claim that bodyweight training is inadequate for building strong legs.

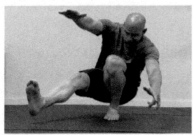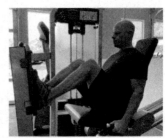

Too little stability can make strength training inefficient, but too much can make it less "functional."

Thankfully, I learned firsthand how improving stability and mobility were the keys to building stronger legs. Like many others, I was skeptical about building my legs with bodyweight training. I firmly believed that the back squat was the undisputed king for building leg strength when I started calisthenics. I figured that doing progressive bodyweight training would compromise my leg strength. I figured I might maintain my little leg strength and muscle at best. At first, my perception seemed valid as I stumbled and struggled with traditional progressive lower body calisthenics. Nothing I did left me feeling like I had satisfyingly worked my legs. That all changed when I started to apply my progressive squat techniques to a set of suspension straps.

As with upper body training, suspension straps expand your potential to progress and regress your lower body exercises. The great thing is that progressive variability extends beyond just the amount of resistance on your legs; it also changes the stability and mobility requirements. These features give you much more control over the difficulty of the exercise, so you can customize it to be the perfect level for you and your abilities.

The straps also allow you to address imbalances and weaknesses that may be holding your lower body strength in check, both with calisthenics and weight lifting. So even if you make weighted leg work your main leg-day staple, you'll still level up your workouts by supplementing them with suspension squat-chain exercises.

Here are some basic guidelines to help you get the most out of your training.

Use Triple Flexion whenever possible

Most coaches recognize that the basic squat movement pattern involves triple extension, extending the ankle, knee, and hip as you stand upright. Unfortunately, the emphasis on triple flexion is seldom addressed.

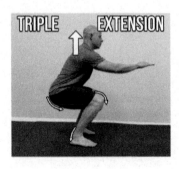 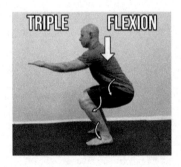

Triple flexion helps balance all squatting movement patterns and significantly reduces your joints' stress. It also improves stability and mobility in your lower body while building strength. The key is to imagine pulling yourself into the squat. Think about pulling your knees forward as you sit on the back of your shoes as you descend to the bottom of each repetition. This emphasis will help engage the muscles in your shin, hamstrings, and hip flexors, enabling that triple flexion. It can take a little practice, but the motion should make your squat feel more natural and comfortable.

Imaging closing the gap between your hips and heels

When I started my coaching career, I used the common queue of telling clients to squat as if sitting back in a chair. This queue works very well for the first half of the movement, but it is possible to overdo it and throw too much of your weight back towards your heels. This technique can result in a relatively unstable and unnatural movement pattern for the lower body.

Instead, I encourage you to start the movement by moving your hips back but continue with pulling your hips closer to your heels. This arching motion increases the mobility in your hips and ankles.

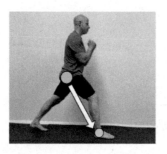 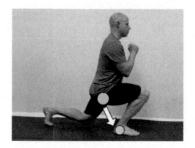

Moving in this way is also particularly handy for lunges and single-leg exercises that can otherwise be problematic if you push your weight too far back.

It's okay to round your back

Flexing the spine as you descend into a squat is one of the cardinal sins in weightlifting, but it's not that bad for bodyweight training. In some cases, it may be unavoidable and maybe even beneficial.

The concern over rounding the back is certainly justified when you have a heavy load on your upper body, like during a back squat or holding a heavy weight. With suspension training, such loading on the body isn't present, so there's not as much need to maintain a perfectly flat back. Holding onto the suspension handles also provides support for the lower back.

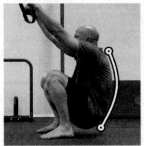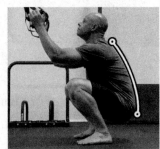

Letting the back round with suspension calisthenics is okay, but keep the arch minimal to improve posture and weight distribution.

You'll still want to minimize the curvature in the spine over time, not for safety reasons but simply because it makes the squat exercise a bit more challenging and a more strict technique. But don't worry if your back has some slight curvature as you descend into your squat. After all, the spine is like any other joint structure in the body; it's healthy to keep it moving and mobile.

Keep your foot and knee on your centerline

This rule applies to unilateral exercises where you work one leg at a time. When you place most of your weight on one leg, it's important to maintain lateral stability by keeping your foot and knee close to the centerline of your body. This tilting and twisting of the hips can produce stress misalignment in your joints and make it difficult to work your lower body.

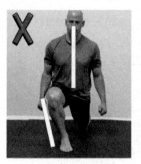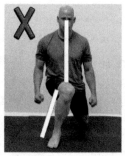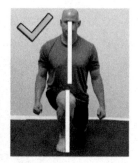

Keeping your foot on your centerline will also require more strength and mobility in your lateral hip. Your thigh will also have a slight inward angle which is perfectly normal and natural. As long as your knee still drives forward over your toes, there shouldn't be any undue stress on your knee joint. If you notice any strain on your knees, I recommend using a shorter range of motion until your hips become more mobile.

Try to rely on the straps as little as possible

Suspension squat training is one of the rare cases where you want to use the suspension straps as little as possible. You want most of your weight on your legs, so placing weight through your arms and, therefore, into the straps will remove resistance from the muscles you're trying to work.

You could even say that the goal is to eventually graduate to not using the straps and place all your weight on your lower body. The straps are almost like a tool to use less instead of enhancing your training by using them more.

Don't feel you have to rush the process. It's perfectly fine to rely on the straps as much as necessary to dial in your technique and optimize your body position. Using the straps for assistance and support is far more effective if you can use a stronger technique than forgo the straps and practice some half-baked freeform exercises.

Besides, as we'll explore here, some more challenging squatting variations can use the straps to adopt a much more difficult squatting technique.

SUSPENSION SQUATS

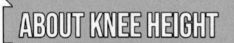

ABOUT KNEE HEIGHT

NARROW OR SHOULDER WIDTH

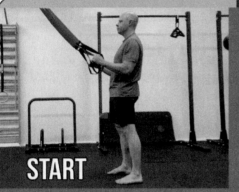

START

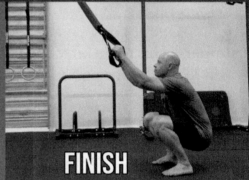

FINISH

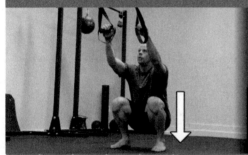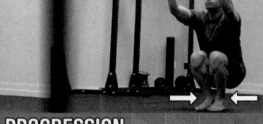

PROGRESSION

NOTES:

Suspension squats are the perfect opportunity to work on perfecting your technique. Be sure to keep your heels down with your weight just to the front of your heel. Look up to the anchor point and drive your ups up and forward when standing up. Be sure your knees track right over your toes and do your best not to lean back against the straps.

Most progression is achieved by increasing the depth of your hips, and you can also move your feet inward to prepare your legs for more advanced squat techniques to come.

REVERSE LUNGES

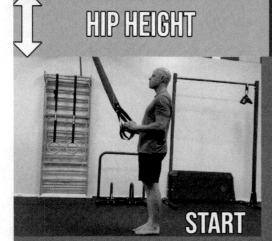

HIP HEIGHT

START

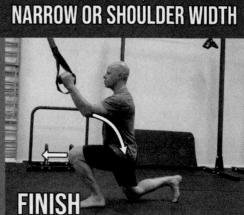

NARROW OR SHOULDER WIDTH

FINISH

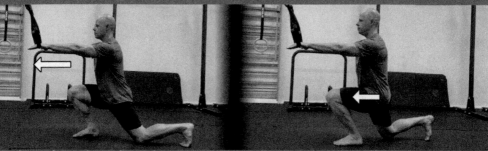

PROGRESSION

NOTES:

Reverse lunges introduce you to unilateral squat techniques that place more weight on one leg. These are a "lunge" but do your best to keep your weight on the front leg. Imagine these are single leg squats with assistance on the back leg. Keep your knee tracking over your front toes and torso only slightly bent forward at the hips.

You can progress by shifting more weight onto the front squatting leg and by extending your arms out in front of you so your arms have less leverage. I like to place my hands in the foot slings to ensure they don't grab and pull too much on the handles.

REAR ELEVATED SPLIT SQUATS (RESS)

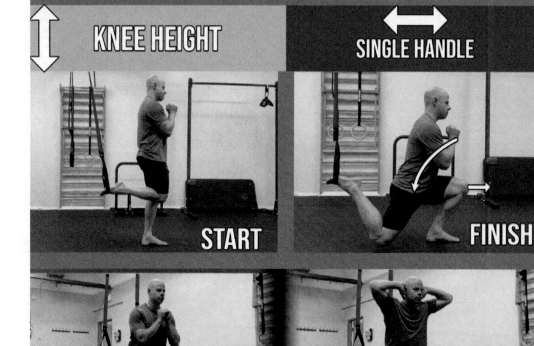

KNEE HEIGHT

START

SINGLE HANDLE

FINISH

PROGRESSION

NOTES:

RESS are the same movement pattern as rev. lunges, but further challenge your mobility and stability. I recommend keeping something near by you can place a hand on in case you lose your balance. Do your best to treat these as a single leg squat with rear leg assistance and don't let the rear foot reach too far back.

Progression is once again achieved by squatting deeper and keeping more weight on the front foot. You can also bring your hands behind your head "prisoner style" to make yourself a bit more top-heavy which increases the demand on the front leg.

PISTOL SQUATS

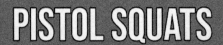

KNEE HEIGHT

NARROW OR SHOULDER WIDTH

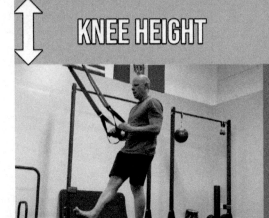

START

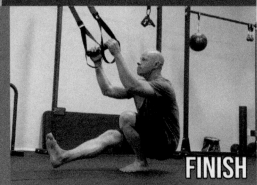

FINISH

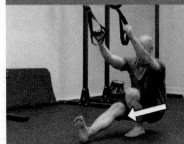

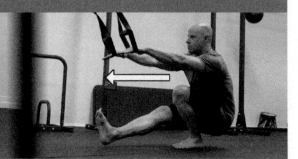

PROGRESSION

NOTES:

Suspension pistol squats allow for more control and stability than unsupported pistol squats making them safer and more effective. These are one of the deepest squat techniques in suspension calisthenics so watch out for the tendency to fall back into the bottom of the squat.

The best way to progress this technique is to pull yourself onto your squatting foot as much as possible so you have less weight on your hands. You can also extend your arms out while placing your palms on the foot loops to take weight off your hands.

HOVER LUNGES

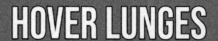

KNEE HEIGHT

NARROW OR SHOULDER WIDTH

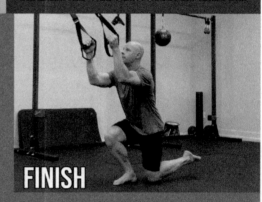

START **FINISH**

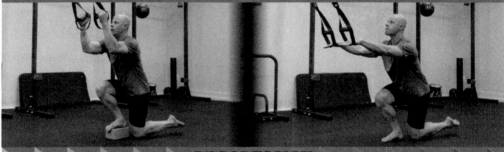

PROGRESSION

NOTES:

Hover lunges place a lot of leverage directly on your front squatting leg while also providing a bit of an isometric hamstring curl. Be sure not to let the back foot touch the floor at all as it may provide a bit of assistance in the squat. As always, try to keep as much weight on your squatting leg as possible with only light assistance through your arms. Do your best not to lean your torso forward too much as you squat. Ideally, your spine and front shin should be at the same angle.

Progress this technique by either standing on an elevated surface to increase the depth of your squat or extend your arms. You can also do both for a real hard squat challenge.

Second level squat chain exercises

As with second-level push and pull chain exercises, second-level squat chain techniques break down the general movement pattern into several single-joint exercises.

Use these as supplemental exercises which are suitable for warm-ups or finishers. However, I've long found the sissy squat and hamstring curls to be quite effective in enhancing the legs' strength and muscle mass. If you have trouble making the squat movement pattern work for you, you might find some value in focusing on these exercises for a couple of months to build up any weak links in your lower body. They can be quite humbling yet also satisfying for your leg workouts.

Don't forget to be mindful of your weight distribution between your upper and lower body. Placing more weight on your hands will typically remove weight, and therefore resistance, on your working leg muscles.

SISSY SQUATS

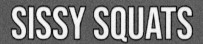

KNEE HEIGHT

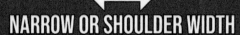

NARROW OR SHOULDER WIDTH

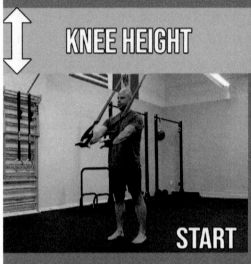

START   FINISH

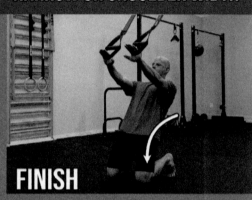

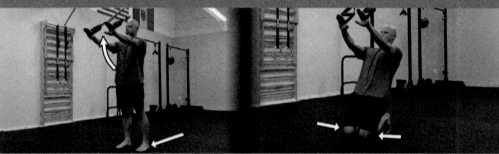

PROGRESSION

NOTES:

Suspension sissy squats are bodyweight leg extensions which place a lot of emphasis on your quads. The key is to keep your glutes and hamstrings tense to lock your hips. Keep the arms straight as you push your knees forward and down toward the floor. Pause at the bottom and use your quads to stand back up while keeping your hips tight.

The primary way to progress is to step forward which raises your arms and forces more of your weight back as you lower your knees down. You can also progress with a more narrow stance.

HAMSTRING CURLS

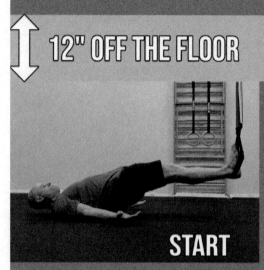

⬍ 12" OFF THE FLOOR

START

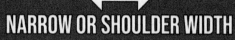

↔ NARROW OR SHOULDER WIDTH

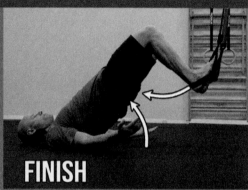

FINISH

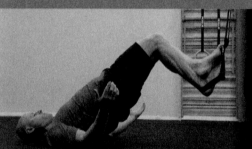

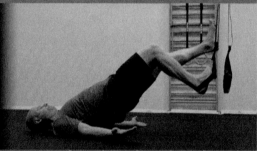

▶▶▶▶▶ PROGRESSION ▷▷▷▷▷

NOTES:

Suspension hamstring curls are one of the most complete hamstring exercises in existence. The trick is to keep your entire posterior chain tense and locked, especially your hips, so you stay stiff as a board as you pull your heels under you. Do your best not to hinge at your hips as you pull in. Also keep your shoulders packed down and tight to have a stable point to pivot on.

Progress by using just one strap and crossing one ankle on top of the other. You can even do single leg curls for the ultimate challenge.

CALF RAISES

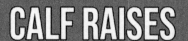

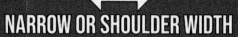

KNEE HEIGHT

NARROW OR SHOULDER WIDTH

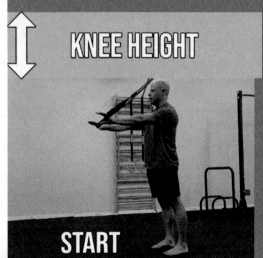

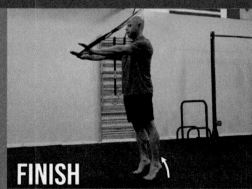

START

FINISH

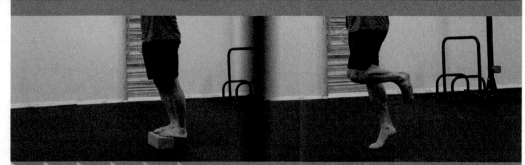

PROGRESSION

NOTES:

Suspension calf raises are just like normal standing calf rasies, where the straps can provide some support and assistance. Try not to lean on your hands so you keep as much weight on the balls of your feet as possible. Keep your glutes, quads, and hamstrings tense to lock your knees and hips in place.

Progress this technique just as you would classic standing calf raises by either standing on an elevated surface to increase your range of motion and/or use one leg at a time.

HIP SWEEPS

HIP HEIGHT
NARROW OR SHOULDER WIDTH

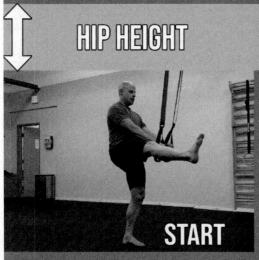

START

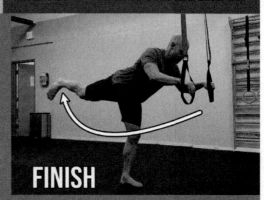

FINISH

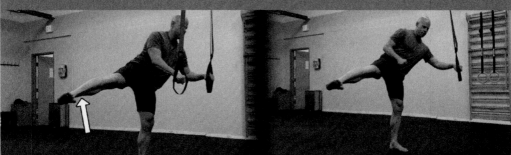

PROGRESSION

NOTES:

Hip sweeps use all of your hip to swing one leg from straight in front of you to pointing behind you in a smooth motion. Try to keep your leg up and locked straight all the way around from front to back before swinging it back to the front again. You'll notice the hip of your standing leg is also working and being stretched as well.

The two best ways to progress this technique are to work on lifting the leg higher, or you can hold onto one handle to challenge your stability.

#5

Flexion Chain Exercises

One of the first gyms I ever worked at had a small weight room that looked like it came right out of Pumping Iron. The weight room had loads of old-school free weights and simple cable machines built during the golden age of bodybuilding. The simple equipment appealed to the more hard-core members, but this was back in the early 2000s. At that time, any decent gym had to have the latest high-tech weight machines, not to mention a collection of ab machines.

It wasn't uncommon for new gyms to have an entire area dedicated to "core" training machines and gadgets. Of course, those over-built lumbar-destroying machines seldom did anything to build a truly strong core. They were also pretty useless for timing away belly fat. Even so, gym managers loved those machines because they looked cool and gave prospective members the impression that their gym was cutting edge. The humble iron pit I worked at appeared to be quite old-fashioned when offering such amenities.

That all changed when I received my first set of Jungle Gym XT suspension straps and hung them from the frame of the cable crossover machine. Just like that, we had a do-it-all ab machine.

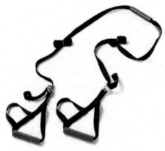

The original Jungle Gym XT was the first ab machine in the free weight gym.

Of course, a lot of members didn't share in my enthusiasm. That simple length of nylon and plastic handles didn't look as fancy as a $3K Cybex weight machine, let alone a collection of such machines. However, even the toughest skeptics quickly adopted the Jungle Gym once they experienced a few of the following exercises, provided they also observed the following key points.

Use your entire flexion chain

While most of these techniques are "abdominal" exercises, don't forget that you're trying to engage and work your entire flexion chain. Don't try to isolate your abs; work them with your hip flexors, quads, and shin muscles.

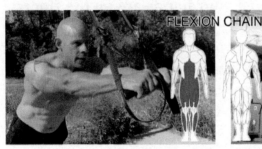
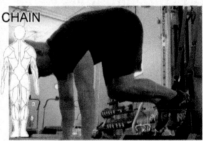

Be mindful of your pelvic tilt

Many abdominal exercises use a great deal of flexion in the hips to bend your body in half, but your abs provide relatively little motion while using those techniques. Instead, your abs are mostly responsible for creating and controlling the tilt of your pelvis. Unfortunately, many people have a lot of difficulties creating a strong pelvic tilt, which is why most people fail to get much from their abdominal training.

I recommend warming up for your flexion chain training with the classic "Cat-Cow" yoga exercise, where you practice creating an anterior and posterior pelvic tilt. Be sure to squeeze your abs as tight as possible with a posterior tilt, as that's the primary job your abs perform in most flexion chain exercises.

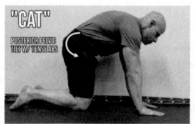 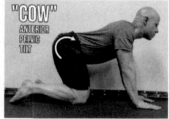

Protract your shoulders when your hands are on the floor

Stable shoulders are an ultra-important aspect of many flexion chain suspension exercises. Protracting your shoulders supports the upper body and provides a stronger foundation for creating the posterior pelvic tilt while doing planks.

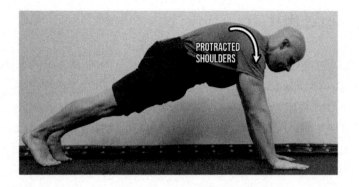

Use your glutes

It may seem strange, but your glutes and hamstrings also play a vital role in helping you build strong abs. Those muscles extend your hips, which can work synergistically with your abs to create that all-important pelvic tilt.

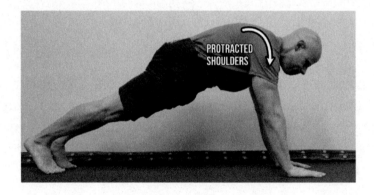

It is true, as they say, that the key to building the muscles in the front of the body is to engage and strengthen the muscles in the back. Nowhere is this more true than using the glutes to develop the abs.

Don't do things that strain your lower back

Lower back strain is one of the most common issues people face when doing core-focused exercises. Many people resort to supporting their hips with their hands, like while doing leg raises, or they simply struggle through the discomfort and accept it as a cost to their ab training. Both of these approaches are big mistakes that will hold you back.

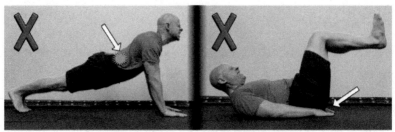

You may be able to continue holding the plank or doing leg raises, but sagging or using your hands for support means your abs are no longer getting a good workout.

Lower back stress during flexion exercises has a simple cause; weak abdominals. Many abdominal exercises use your hip flexors, including your Psoas muscle. Your psoas muscle runs from your femur, through your pelvis, and has many attachment points along your lumbar spine.

Flexing your hip causes your psoas to fire and pull against your lower back. Normally, this pulling is perfectly fine and doesn't cause any issue, just as long as your abdominals can contract with enough tension to balance out the force in your lumbar spine.

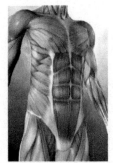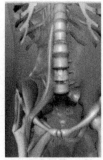

Both the Rectus Abdominis (left) and Psoas Major (right) play a role in most flexion chain exercises. The key is to use both to maintain a balance of force in your lower back.

Some coaches try to mitigate the issue by bypassing the activation of the hip flexors to "isolate" the abdominals. Not only is the action completely unnatural, but it can hold the strength of your flexion chain in check. Your abs and hip flexors should work together whenever you flex your hip for anything from walking and stepping to kicking and even squatting.

Feeling stress in your lower back shows that your abdominals are not strong enough and fail to support your lumbar spine. Trying to shut off your hip flexors is not only unnecessary; it can even enable your abdominals to stay weak.

You want to focus on using exercise variations, where you can create a very high amount of tension in your abdominals and total control in your pelvis. You should feel your abs working very hard with all of these exercises. If you feel it in your lower back, stop the set and rest or regress to an easier exercise.

Prioritize intensity over volume

Volume is a common point of pride when it comes to abdominal training. Core workouts can often involve endless reps and sets or holding isometric positions, like a plank, for several minutes. Some people use so much volume that they dedicate entire workouts to just working their abs.

High-volume work can feel satisfying, but flexion chain training depends on the same principles for any muscle group. Volume and intensity are inversely related. If you have more of one, you have less of the other. The more you prioritize volume, the more you compromise the intensity of muscle tension.

There's a time and place for all forms of training, but I've long observed that athletes gain more benefit by prioritizing intensity over volume. I've selected some of my favorite suspension exercises that can thoroughly work your flexion chain in under ten repetitions or 15-20 seconds. The leverage of these exercises makes achieving such intensity supremely efficient and safe making these techniques some of the best abdominal training exercises in existence.

SUSPENSION PLANK

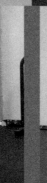 **6" ABOVE FLOOR** | **NARROW OR SHOULDER WIDTH**

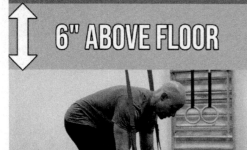

START | **FINISH**

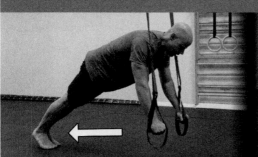 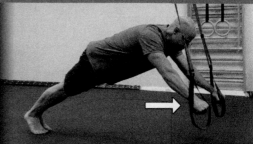

PROGRESSION

NOTES:

Suspension planks are one of the simplest ways to work your flexion chain and work your abdominals with a lot of intensity. Start with your weight on your feet and reach your arms out to straighten your body in a controlled fashion. Hold for time while maintaining tension in your abs, glutes and lats. Keep the straps about an inch from the top of your shoulders.

Progress by moving yourself back which places more weight on your hands. You can also increase the resistance by reaching your arms out in front of you a few inches.

FOOT SUSPENSION PLANK

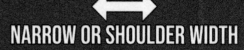

FOOT LOOPS ABOUT 12" ABOVE FLOOR

NARROW OR SHOULDER WIDTH

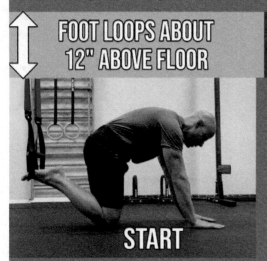

START

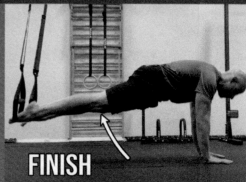

FINISH

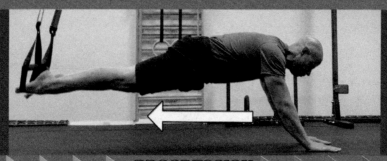

PROGRESSION

NOTES:

Foot suspension planks are a bit more challenging than regular suspension planks partly because they start you on the floor and elevate your feet. Begin with your knees on the floor and tilt your pelvis to engage your abs. Pick up your knees into the plank position and hold for time. Be sure to maintain tension in your glutes and protract your shoulders.

The primary way to progress this technique is to shift yourself back. You can shift back and hold or perform a "saw plank" where you shift back and forth for reps.

KNEE-TUCKS/PIKE-UPS

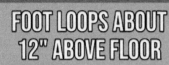

FOOT LOOPS ABOUT 12" ABOVE FLOOR

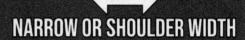

NARROW OR SHOULDER WIDTH

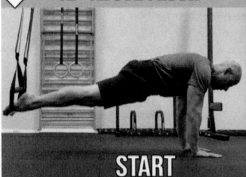

START

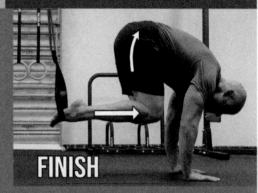

FINISH

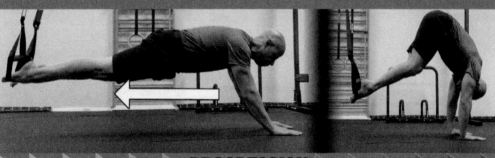

PROGRESSION

NOTES:

Knee-tucks and pike-ups are more dynamic variations of foot suspension planks where you pull your knees up towards you chest while lifting your hips. They are not only a great way to work your flexion chain, but they also improve the mobility of your extension chain as well so strive for as much range of motion with each repetition.

You can progress these by shifting your weight back, just as you would with foot planks at the bottom of each rep, or you can keep your legs straighter in a "pike-up."

LYING LEG RAISES

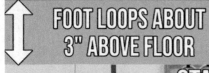

FOOT LOOPS ABOUT 3" ABOVE FLOOR

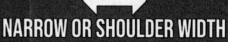

NARROW OR SHOULDER WIDTH

START   **FINISH**

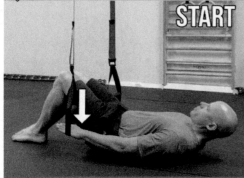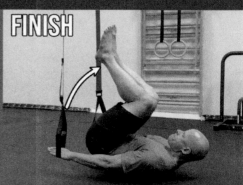

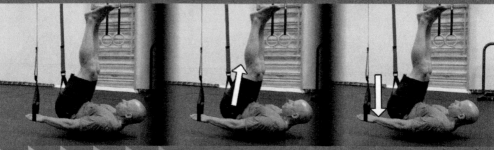

PROGRESSION

NOTES:

Suspension lying leg raises are just like normal lying leg raises, but you're pressing your hands down onto the handles or foot loops to increase resistance and improve stability. Start lying on the floor with your shoulders slightly elevated off the ground and press down to engage your abs. Maintain downward pressure as you tuck your pelvis upward to lift your legs.

Progression with the exercise is mostly achieved by straightening your legs, but you can also increase resistance by lifting your hips up higher and pressing down harder.

SUSPENSION SIT-UPS

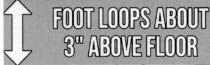 **FOOT LOOPS ABOUT 3" ABOVE FLOOR**

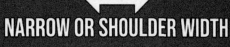 **NARROW OR SHOULDER WIDTH**

START **FINISH**

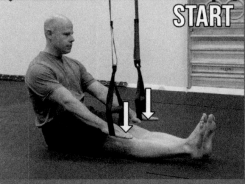 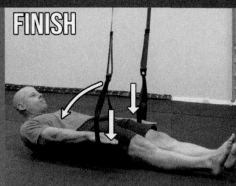

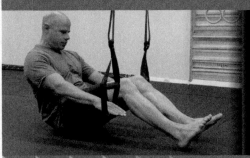 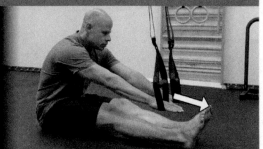

▶ ▶ ▶ ▶ ▶ PROGRESSION

NOTES:

Suspension sit-ups are also a more stable, yet challenging variation on a classic abdominal exercise. Start in the top position and firmly press down into the foot straps. Continue to press down as you sit back onto the floor. Maintain downward pressure as you pause at the bottom and then sit back up again.

Progression is primarily achieved by pressing down harder onto the straps, but you can also bend your knees to make the exercise more challenging. You can also strive to reach forward more at the top of each repetition.

SUSPENSION L-SIT

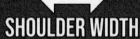

KNEE HEIGHT

SHOULDER WIDTH

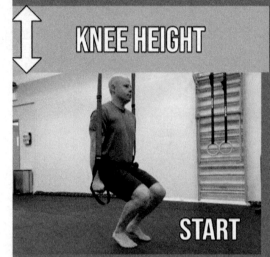

START

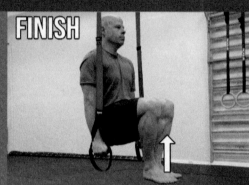

FINISH

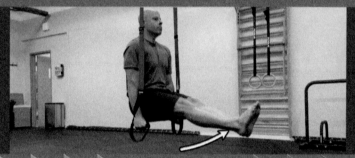

PROGRESSION

NOTES:

The classic L-sit is a true total body exercise, and doing them on suspension straps makes them even more so. The key to working your abs harder is to use your back muscles as much as possible especially your lats. The more you engage your lats, the more you can push your hips forward and create a posterior pelvic tilt.

Progression is primarily achieved by extending the legs out in front of you, with more extension offering more resistance. You can also continue to push your pelvis forward as much as you can to increase resistance as well.

KNEE/LEG RAISE

WAIST HEIGHT

SHOULDER WIDTH

START

FINISH

PAUSE

PROGRESSION

NOTES:

Knee raises are the dynamic variation of the L-sit so the same principles apply including using the back for stability. Moving the legs up and down increases the challenge to the abs while also requiring more stability from the back as well. Try to moving in a smooth and controlled motion to avoid momentum taking over and making the exercise easier.

Progression is achieved in the same manner as the L-Sit where you extend the legs out to increase resistance. You can also make this technique more difficult by trying to lift the legs higher and pausing at the top for a full second.

HANGING LEG RAISE

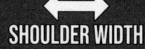

OVERHEAD REACH

SHOULDER WIDTH

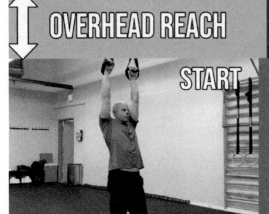

START   FINISH

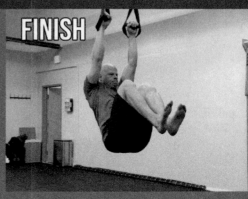

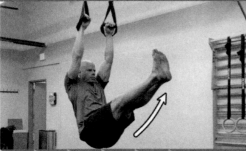

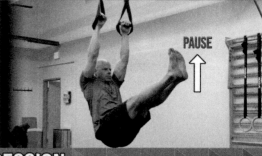

PAUSE

PROGRESSION

NOTES:

The hanging knee/leg raise is fundamentally the same exercise as the classic knee raise, only now you're hanging from the handles at an overhead reach position. In some ways, this may be easier than holding yourself in place than with the handles at waist height, but it can also be more challenging on the grip and shoulder muscles. Once again, be sure to use your whole back for stability and try to use your upper back to push your torso forward as you lift your legs.

The progression strategy is the same as with the previous leg raise where extending your legs and pausing at the top are the main ways to make the exercise more challenging.

#6

Extension Chain Exercises

The extension or posterior chain is one of the most important areas of the body you can work. It includes all of the muscles along your backside, and these exercises will focus on the muscles that extend the hips and spine.

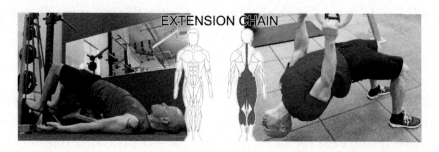

Whenever I start to coach suspension extension exercises, I recall an incident when I felt like my right hamstring was getting torn in half.

Years ago, I made an annual tradition of participating in the infamous Vermont 50 mountain bike race. As the name implies, the event was a 50-mile loop in southern Vermont that finished on the Mt. Ascutney ski resort.

The race was always a fun adventure, except that I tended to suffer nagging hamstring cramps toward the end of the race. Usually, the cramping was little more than a recurring nuisance, but one year the cramps started to come on with very high intensity. The cramping became so bad that I had trouble walking on flat ground.

I did my best to drink water and take electrolyte pills, but my hamstrings worsened as the day went on. I was riding a stretch of single track and hit a rock that forced me to step down off my bike. When my foot hit the ground, my entire hamstring was cramped with excruciating intensity. I immediately fell into the brush, but the impact worsened the cramp. My whole hamstring continued to cramp up tighter and tighter. It felt like someone was slowly stabbing a knife in my leg. All I could do was just lay there in agony and hope the cramp would pass. When it eventually did, I wasn't sure if I could walk, let alone ride the rest of the race. Thankfully, I could finish the race but not without a great deal of discomfort.

That incident left me with a strong motivation to solve my cramping issue once and for all. I knew things like hydration and nutrition were key, but I was already addressing those variables to the point of overkill, so I knew that wasn't the ultimate solution. The only other option was to make my hamstrings more resilient through strength training.

Most of my lower body training at the time was nothing more than heavy back squats. I was doing very little to train my glutes and hamstrings directly. Since I was in the free-weights-are-best phase of my training career, I made deadlifts, kettlebell swings, and my posterior chain bread and butter for the next several years.

Focusing on building up my hamstrings worked, but only to a point. I was still cramping up, but I could ride longer before the cramping started, and the cramps were less severe. I just figured I was one of those folks who had cramp-happy hamstrings.

I held that belief until I attended a one-day TRX instructor seminar. I was comfortable with most upper body exercises but never explored suspension lower body training. I figured nothing could match heavy lifting, so I never bothered with it. Boy, was I in for a surprise! We started with "light" TRX hip extensions, and my hamstrings went crazy on the first repetition. I never knew my hamstrings could work that hard. It wasn't just the intensity that lit my hammies up like Times Square; it was the holistic nature of the exercises. Until then, I focused solely on hip extension-based exercises like romanian deadlifts. The suspension hamstring techniques worked every muscle fiber along the back of my legs. Even my calves and the muscles in the bottom of my feet were working hard.

Since then, I've made suspension hamstring and posterior chain exercises a staple of my training and for the clients I coach. My cramping issues have since become a thing of the past. Plus, my hamstrings are far more active with everything I do, from kicking and running to simply walking and even standing up from a chair.

One of the great things about suspension hamstring work is that they are almost fool-proof. It's almost impossible not to work your glutes and hamstrings with the following exercises. It takes skill and muscle activation to work your hamstrings with free weights, but suspension extension exercises make it easier to work the entire hamstring complex. These tips will help you get more out of the exercises in this chapter.

Keep your shoulders packed

While much stability comes from your hips, your shoulder blades also support your extension chain. Keeping your shoulder blades down and back ensures you transfer energy along your spine and into your hips. Packing your shoulders also helps prevent stress in your lower back.

Packing your shoulders can take some practice, but it's as simple as pinching the floor with your shoulder blades. In some exercises, pinching your shoulders down and back should slightly lift your chest and may even lift your tailbone off the floor.

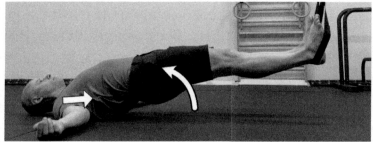

"Packing" the shoulders down helps pull the torso into a slight arch which also helps elevate the hips off the floor.

Packing your shoulders will also ensure most of the movement comes from your hips and knee flexion, so you drive as much attention as possible into your glutes and hamstrings.

Use both your "lower" and "upper" hamstrings at all times

Your hamstrings effectively have two jobs to fulfill. One job is to flex your knee, while the other is to extend your hip. Using each action employs your entire hamstring complex, but it may be helpful to think of engaging your upper hamstrings, which extend your hip and lower hamstrings that flex your knee.

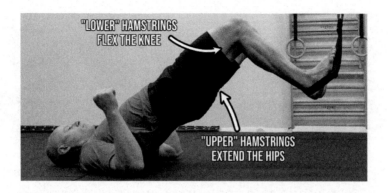

Technically you don't have upper and lower hamstrings since most of them run the entire length of your thigh, yet it can help to imagine what joint you're trying to emphasize with some exercises.

Almost all extension chain exercises will require engaging both your knee and hip activation. While you may not move at both joints, you'll want to engage the hamstrings to stabilize your knees and hips.

Extend your spine, but don't pinch your lower back

Slightly extending your spine, especially your thoracic spine, can be very helpful in ensuring you maintain a packed set of shoulder blades while also reducing stress in the lumbar spine.

Feeling a pinch or stress in the lower back indicates that your upper back isn't working to stabilize your shoulders or that your glutes and hamstrings are not engaged enough to stabilize your hips. Also, just as keeping your glutes tight can help you engage your abs, you may now find that engaging your abs can help you engage your glutes.

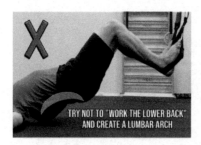 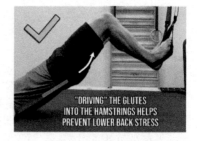

TRY NOT TO "WORK THE LOWER BACK" AND CREATE A LUMBAR ARCH

"DRIVING" THE GLUTES INTO THE HAMSTRINGS HELPS PREVENT LOWER BACK STRESS

Trying to extend your spine fully does wonders to ensure this doesn't happen while also engaging your spinal erectors.

Before jumping into the primary suspension extension chain exercises, I left out the suspension hamstring curls because I already included them in the squat chain chapter. Hamstring curls are both an extension and squat chain technique due to the hamstrings' role in most leg exercises. So feel free to include them in your extension chain workouts if you like; they work well for that purpose.

SUSPENSION BRIDGE

⬍ WAIST HEIGHT

⬌ SHOULDER WIDTH

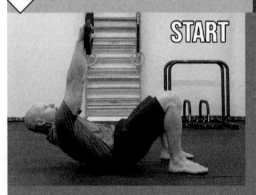

START

FINISH

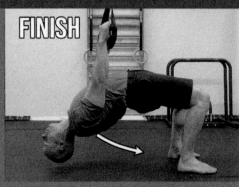

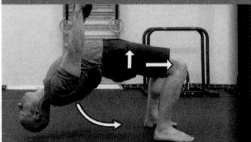

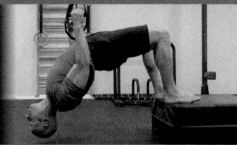

▶ ▶ ▶ ▶ ▶ PROGRESSION ◀ ◀ ◀ ◀ ◀

NOTES:

Suspension bridges are very similar to the classic floor bridge, only now you pull with your arms above the torso on suspension handles instead of pressing off the floor. This change can make the full bridge more accessible for those with limited shoulder and back mobility. These are also a great way to practice the pulling action of your extension chain by making it easier to pull your shoulders back toward your heels.

Most progression is accomplished by increasing range of motion in the back and hips to create a more rounded back bridge. You can also enhance the challenge by placing your feet on an elevated surface.

SUSPENSION HIP EXT.

KNEE HEIGHT

NARROW OR SHOULDER WIDTH

START

FINISH

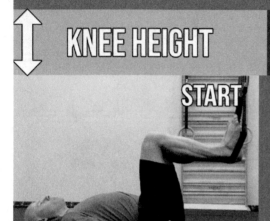
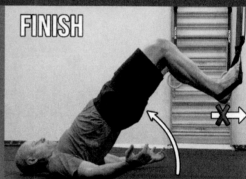

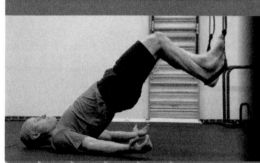
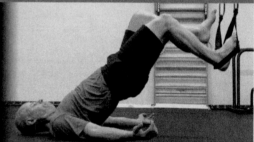

PROGRESSION

NOTES:

Hip extensions are one of the most effective ways to focus on the hip extension aspect of your extension chain. Start with your hips and knees at roughly a 90-degree angle and lift your hips by driving the back of your heels into the foot straps. Do your best to not push the feet forward as you lift up.

This exercise is sort of the opposite of hamstring curls. With curls, you lock your hips and move at the knee joint. With these you lock the knee joint and move at the hips. This means you can progress the technique in the same ways with increasing ROM, crossing ankles and using single-leg variations.

SUSPENSION HIP BRIDGE

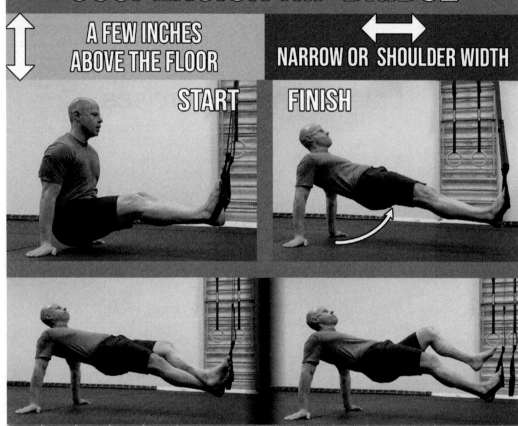

A FEW INCHES ABOVE THE FLOOR

NARROW OR SHOULDER WIDTH

START

FINISH

PROGRESSION

NOTES:

These hip bridges are a great gut-check exercise to identify how well you can coordinate tension throughout your extension chain. While you drive the hips up and forward, these will not be possible if you also don't keep tension throughout your hamstrings and along your spine. Be sure to also keep your shoulders packed down tight.

As with the other hip extension exercises, progression is made through increasing range of motion and progressing to a cross ankle and then single-leg variations. You can also play with placing your hands further forward or back to slightly modify the leverage against the straps.

#7

Lateral Chain Exercises

Lateral chain exercises and workouts are not the most popular tension chain to work. Many people prefer to skip the exercises in this chapter entirely. This lack of focus is fine since you're already working all of your lateral chain muscles with the other exercises.

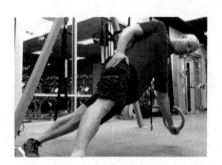

LATERAL CHAIN

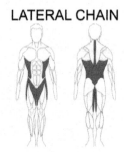

These exercises are not about working the muscles per se but rather to help you engage the muscles as a complete unit so they can provide support along the sides of the body. The goal here is to "knit" the tension in the muscles together, which will help with twisting, throwing, kicking, and total body stability.

These exercises are pretty simple, and they largely rely on using the body in an isometric fashion. However, some movements can strengthen your lateral chain, like twisting or lateral lifting. Here are several key points to keep in mind when training your lateral chain.

Maintain tension along your entire lateral chain

Lateral chain training often focuses on targeting the obliques or the hips. This approach isn't incorrect; it is also important to include all of the other muscles along the chain to facilitate a complete transfer force along the side of your body.

There's nothing wrong with feeling an emphasis on the hips or obliques. Just be sure to still engage your lats, shoulders, and the lateral muscles in the thigh, including your quadriceps and hamstrings.

Avoid folding at the hips and retract your shoulders.

Folding at the hips and hunching forward are two of the most common mistakes people make with lateral training.

These discrepancies are not necessarily dangerous, but they do substantially reduce your stability and remove effective tension from the muscles you are trying to target.

That's why lateral exercises are also extension chain techniques. By fully retracting your shoulders, extending your spine, and pushing the hips forward, you'll ensure a fully engaged lateral chain that helps maintain your stability.

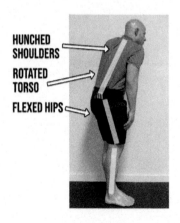
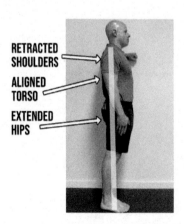

HUNCHED SHOULDERS
ROTATED TORSO
FLEXED HIPS

RETRACTED SHOULDERS
ALIGNED TORSO
EXTENDED HIPS

Work both sides evenly

Lateral chain training is usually practiced one side at a time, so it's crucial to ensure you have an equal stimulus on both sides. Be sure to work both sides of your body at the same level of intensity for the same duration of time.

It is very common to feel like one side is stronger than the other. This discrepancy is not necessarily a bad thing, nor is it a sign of a problematic muscle imbalance. The human body is not supposed to be perfectly ambidextrous, so it's not necessarily bad to feel stronger on one side. However, do your best to ensure both sides are working as equally as possible. If one side feels like it's all in the hips and the other side feels like it's on the shoulders, take that as an opportunity to check your position and technique to ensure you are using both sides the same way.

F.S. SIDE PLANK

12" ABOVE THE FLOOR

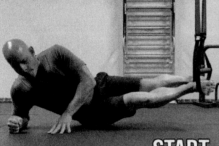

START

NARROW OR SHOULDER WIDTH

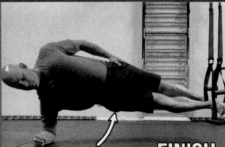

FINISH

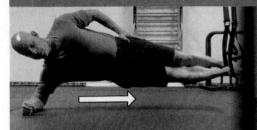

▶ ▶ ▶ ▶ ▶ PROGRESSION

NOTES:

The foot suspended side plank is a bread and butter lateral chain exercise. Placing your feet in the foot slings removed a point of contact with the floor and requires more strength in your muscles. Start with your hips on the floor and press your feet sideways into the straps. Use your hand to assist if necessary. Hold for time and repeat on the other side.

You can progress through moving your hips up and down to make it a dynamic exercise, or push yourself away from your supporting elbow to add resistance. You can combine both motions for even more challenge.

H.S. SIDE PLANK

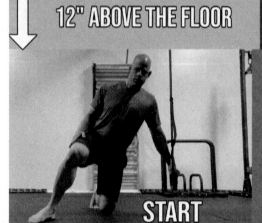

START

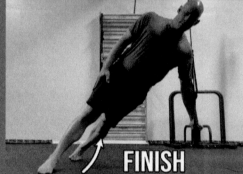

FINISH

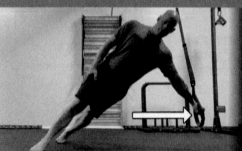

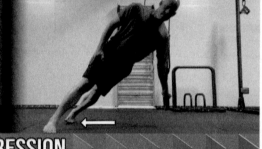

PROGRESSION

NOTES:

The hand suspended side plank places more resistance against the upper body compared to the foot suspended plank. Be sure to fully engage the lats on the side of the support arm and keep the shoulder depressed. Start with the back knee on the floor and lean onto the hand. Lift the back knee up to achieve the plank using a staggered stance.

Progression is mostly achieved by reaching the arm out further to increase resistance or by moving away from the anchor point to place more weight on the hand. You can also make this move more difficult by using a more narrow stance with your feet.

TWISTING PLANK

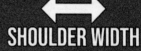

12" ABOVE THE FLOOR

SHOULDER WIDTH

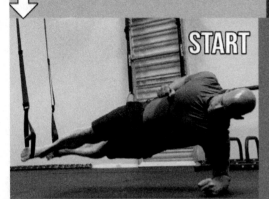

START

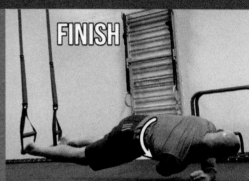

FINISH

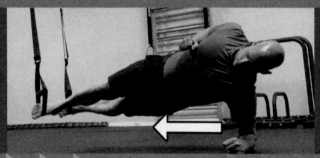

▶▶▶▶▶ PROGRESSION ▷▷▷▷▷

NOTES:

The twisting plank uses the lateral chain, but it's also a fantastic shoulder and scapula stability exercise. I recommend playing with this technique with your feet on the ground first to get the feel for the technique. From there, progress to suspending your feet in the foot slings and allow your feet to rotate within the straps.

Progression is primarily achieved by increasing range of motion in the shoulder while you maintain a stable posture. You can also shift yourself back away from your arm to add resistance onto your lateral chain.

#8

Suspension Mobility Training

One of the most unusual pieces of exercise equipment I've ever used was a cage-like contraption called a True Stretch. It was a large contraption that looked like something you would find at the local playground, with assorted bars and handles to anchor your hands and feet.

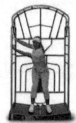 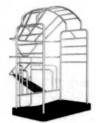 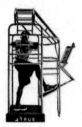

The True Stretch cage made stretching easier compared to plain floor stretches. Photo: Truefitness.com

The premise behind the True Stretch was that stretching on the floor was uncomfortable and ineffective. You didn't have full control of your body position relative to gravity, which compromised your ability to get an effective deep stretch. The cage was designed to give you four supportive points of contact while allowing you to stretch in multiple planes of motion. These advantages were supposed to make stretching safer and more productive.

To be honest, I've never been a big fan of stretching. Despite always doing it before Taekwon-Do class, I've always found it tedious, not to mention not very effective. Stretching never made me feel flexible or any looser during a warm-up. I still pulled muscles while kicking, no matter how much I stretched my legs. Despite my frustration with the practice, I liked using the True Stretch much more than just splaying myself out on the floor. It was much easier to use, and it did help to undo the kinks in my back after sitting in a delivery truck all day. It's just a shame the unit was much too big to fit into my apartment, plus it was far too expensive to be practical for personal use.

Thankfully, I eventually found that I could replicate almost every exercise I did in the True Stretch with simple suspension straps. Full-body control and stability in space? Check! Four points of contact? Check! The ability to decompress the spine and hips? Check! You can have all of the advantages of the True Stretch without the impractical cost.

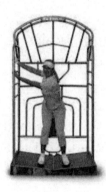 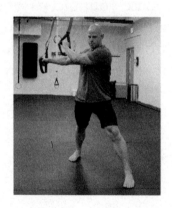

I would even say that stretching on a suspension system can be even more effective since you have the freedom to move your body as you stretch. You have more freedom and movement to dial in every stretch without sacrificing supportive control.

So yes, suspension straps are great for building muscle and strength, but they are also the perfect mobility solution to relieve physical stress. Here are some tips to help you get the most out of your suspension mobility work.

Maintain a bit of tension in the muscles

It may seem a little counterintuitive, but keeping some muscle tension can improve your mobility. You'll achieve a bigger range of motion by relaxing your muscles as much as possible, but keeping some tension in the muscles serves several more important functions.

The first is to improve the tension control in the extended position. It's usually easier to contract a muscle when it's short and flexed; just think of how tense your bicep is when you "make a muscle" and flex your elbow. It's more challenging to maintain some tension in the muscle as it elongates, which is why it's harder to tense your biceps when your arm is straight. Improving tension control in an elongated position improves your physical control throughout a full range of motion, which can help build stronger muscles and helps protect your joints.

Second, a little tension can proactively increase the intensity of the stretch on your muscle fibers. So instead of passively stretching your muscles with a large range of motion, you're slightly shortening your muscle to pull on the muscle proactively.

Lastly, increasing the tension in the muscle can help protect sensitive joints from stress. Stretching is usually pretty joint-friendly, but that doesn't mean it's stress-free. An active muscle is a shock absorber to your joints to handle the forces running through your body. When your muscles are not tense, those forces are still present, and they often are sent straight into your joints.

Breathe throughout the stretch

Breathing is one of the most effective ways to tell your body to be tense and tight or loose and relaxed. While you don't necessarily want to relax fully into a stretch, you don't want to put your body into fight or flight. Continuing to breathe with a slow and smooth breath can help you maintain that sweet spot of having responsive muscles without excessive tension.

One of the most effective breathing techniques for stretching is to release the stretch as you inhale slightly and then push a bit deeper into the stretch as you exhale. Doing so can help you achieve a deeper stretch, but it can also help unify your breathing and tension control, improving your suspension strength training.

Don't worry too much about how long you hold a stretch

As with strength training, the goal of each session isn't just to abide by a numeric formula but to create a stimulus within the muscle. Any variables can influence how long you should practice an exercise, from how warmed-up you are, to tension control and even body position.

So don't worry about holding your stretch for a long time. You should feel like the muscle is starting to stretch out and lengthen during the stretch. Once it's reached that point, you can release the stretch and move on.

Be mindful of your weight distribution

Suspension stretching allows you to have four points of contact, which means you'll distribute your body weight between all four limbs. You'll naturally have most of your weight on the limbs you're stretching out, but keep some weight on the other two to maintain stability and control.

Experiment with your body position during the stretch

Suspension straps allow you to move your body in the stretch, so be playful and experiment with your position in space. There's no perfect or correct way to hold any stretching techniques, so move around and find ways to address the muscles that need it most.

Chest stretch

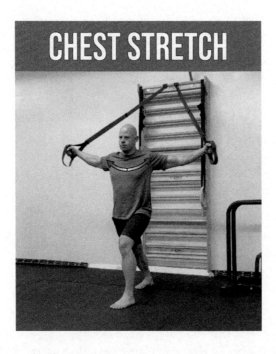

This stretch is one of the best ways to stretch your chest while giving you full control over your body position. Keep your weight on your feet and press your torso forward to allow the straps to pull your hands to the side and slightly behind you. Try not to lean forward, as that might place more weight on your hands and compromise the depth of the stretch. I recommend practicing this with the left and right leg forward to balance the stretch along your torso.

Overhead stretch

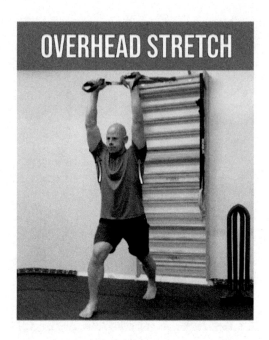

The overhead stretch is the perfect complement to the chest stretch as it stretches out the back and lats, which are often antagonists to the chest muscles. You can also hop right into the stretch from the same body position as the chest stretch; you simply reach your hands overhead and press your torso forward. Try not to arch your back and get as much range as you can through the shoulders.

Standing twist

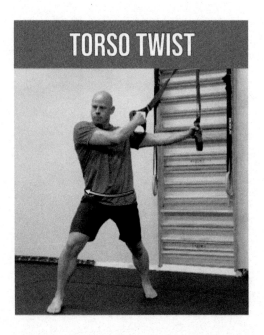

TORSO TWIST

Torso twisting is a great way to explore where you are tight along your lateral chain and hips. It's also a good stretch for the biceps of the rear arm. You can perform this stretch either facing away from the anchor point or side facing it to play around with how you apply force against the body. You may also want to play around with using a lower anchor point to apply the force against the straps in a more lateral direction. This stretch works by holding onto the handles and then twisting your pelvis away from the anchor point. Maintain an upright posture and don't lean against the straps. Be sure to apply this stretch to both sides of the body.

Triceps and back stretch

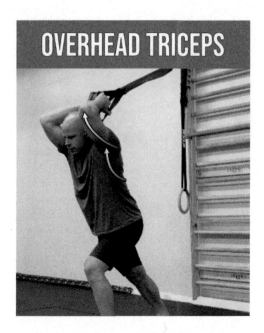

The overhead triceps hit the back the same way as the overhead reach but also stretch the triceps by keeping the elbows bent. Body position is key with this stretch. Keeping your torso upright makes this more of a lat stretch, but hinging forward at the hips will make this more of a triceps stretch. Ensure you keep your weight on your feet to prevent leaning forward too much.

Hamstring hinge

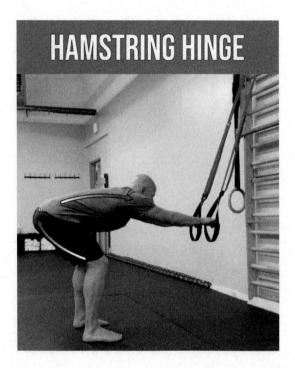

The hamstring hinge is one of my favorite suspension stretches, as it stretches almost every muscle on the backside of the body. It's the perfect compliment to extension chain exercises for this reason. It's also a very versatile stretch with a lot of adjustments you can make to it.

Play around with how much weight you have on your feet versus your hands. Leaning forward will make this a back and shoulder stretch. Leaning back on your feet will place more emphasis on your hamstrings. You can also experiment with keeping your knees straight or letting them bend slightly to adjust the stretch on your hamstrings.

Sit-back stretch

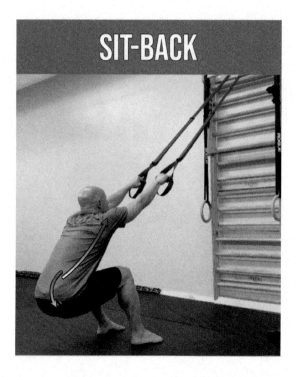

The sit-back stretch is a feel-good exercise that helps decompress the spine and shoulder joint. All you need to do is sit your hips down and back, so most of your weight remains on your hands. Let your hips drop down, and even tuck your pelvis a bit to stretch your lower back. Keeping your torso upright will stretch your upper back more, and dropping your hips helps stretch the lats and lower back. Try twisting the torso slightly from one side to the other to emphasize one side over the other.

Wide shifting squat

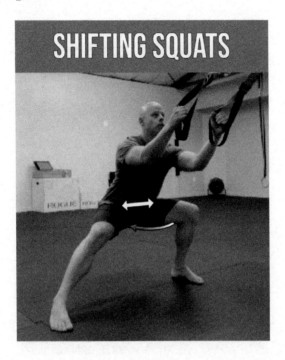

Shifting squats are a great way to work and stretch the adductor muscles inside the hips. Simply get into a wide stance and squat down with your hips returning to place some weight on your hands. Shift your weight from side to side in a smooth and controlled manner to gently stretch the inner thigh. You can also modify this stretch by slightly twisting and tilting your pelvis to change the angle you're stretching.

Figure 4 sit

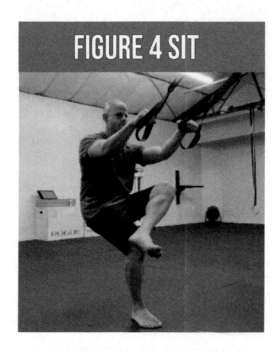

The classic figure 4 sit is the antagonist to the shifting squat and helps stretch the abductors and lateral hip. The deeper you sit, the deeper the stretch will be. It also helps to work the lateral hip to press the knee of the bent leg down toward the floor. You tell from the photo above this is also one of the tightest areas of the body for me, probably due to years of cycling without any lateral hip mobility work.

Wall quad stretch

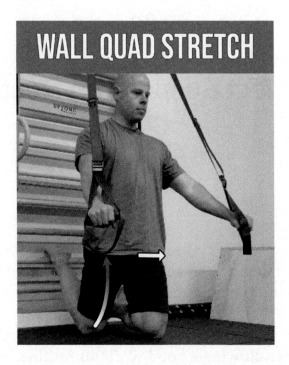

The wall quad stretch involves kneeling on the floor, so you may wish to use a towel or pad for the knees. Place the knee of the quad you wish to stretch closer to the wall with your toes on the wall. Keep equal weight distribution between both knees and your hands as you push your hips forward to stretch the quad. It may also help to slightly lean the torso back. Be sure to repeat on both sides.

#9

The Perfect Suspension Routine For You

We've covered a lot of ground exploring some of the fundamental suspension calisthenics exercises and their variations. Now it's time to show you how to put all those pieces into a plan.

Before we begin, I want to clarify that no one ever achieves their fitness goals by following a good workout routine. However, many people have certainly failed by following a bad one. A good workout routine is like the launchpad for a rocket. It gives you stability and points you in the right direction, but you can't expect any more from it than that. Meanwhile, a bad routine is any sort of plan that makes it difficult to maintain your training consistency or one that encourages you to work toward goals that you don't want.

A successful rocket launch depends on how well the rocket works, just as an effective workout depends on how well your body works. So don't get too hung up on trying to dial in the perfect workout routine. All you need is a plan, any plan at all, that satisfies these key criteria.

#1 Work your muscles according to your goals

Forget the advice you find online about the "best" workout routines to build muscle and strength. Those routines are often based on little more than blind assumptions and guesswork. Besides, you're not going to achieve those goals by following any routine; you achieve them by progressively working your muscles harder. The key is *how* you're working your muscles, which depends on your goals.

Fundamentally, you have two basic variables for working your muscles. The first is how intense your muscles are contracting, and the second is how long they are contracting. Or in simpler terms, time and tension.

There are a million ways to program a strength routine, but they all boil down to adjusting how hard the muscle is working and how long it's working. If you want to emphasize building strength, use exercises that place a lot of tension on the muscle. Program your workouts to emphasize working the muscles for longer periods for stamina and endurance.

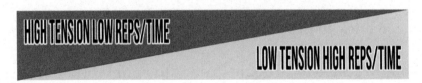

Naturally, both variables come at the expense of the other, but that doesn't mean you can't train for both objectives. You'll simply change your routine, so sometimes, you work with heavier resistances to emphasize building strength and lighter resistance to improve endurance.

When building muscle, you'll generally work with a little of both to give your muscles a broad range of strength and endurance. As long as you're pushing your muscles to a high state of fatigue, you'll create the stimulus for muscle growth.

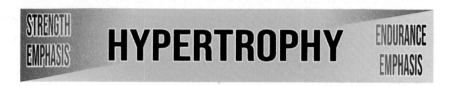

#2 Your routine is somewhat balanced

Calisthenics culture is rife with unbalanced workout routines. Some people spend all their time doing push-ups and pull-ups but seldom work their legs. Others may do hundreds of squats and push-ups but hardly ever work the back of their body.

Using techniques from all six tension chains helps ensure your workouts are well balanced. Don't worry if you have a few more sets or reps in one chain over the other; as long as you have roughly the same amount of work throughout all six chains, you should be fine.

#3 You can stick to the plan with minimal effort

You shouldn't have to struggle to stick to your workout routine. Sure, you'll have momentary lapses in motivation, or life may sometimes get in the way of your training, and that's fine. Aside from instances like that, you should be able to stick to your training without too much effort. Don't be afraid to make whatever changes you feel are necessary to your routine to make your routine easier to maintain.

#4 Change and modify the plan to work for your circumstances

One of the key things that makes a training routine effective is working within your resources and preferences. A two-hour workout routine will be ineffective if you don't have time to practice it. That killer chest routine is no longer an effective plan if you can't hang your straps to do the necessary dips.

So don't be afraid to use a more flexible approach to your routine if it no longer works with your circumstances. If you can't cram a long workout into your busy schedule, plan your workout to fit well within the time you can spend. If you're stuck in your hotel room and can't do dips, change to another challenging pushing exercise you can do in that space.

#5 Prioritize progression over sticking to the routine

I used to pride myself on being a disciplined gym rat who faithfully stuck to a routine no matter what. I did every single workout to the letter no matter what. The only problem was that I did everything "perfectly" in every workout, and nothing changed.

The magic formula for results doesn't come from your routine but from progressively using your muscles over time. If your routine stays the same, then you stay the same. So don't go into your workouts to stick to the routine like a perfectionist. Instead, color outside the lines and look for the changes to level your performance.

This mindset is especially important with suspension calisthenics, where much of your performance is somewhat subjective. Don't be afraid to take an extra step back to add more resistance while doing triceps extensions. Go ahead and crank out a few more rows than you originally planned. Strength isn't so much built as it is discovered. Like any journey of discovery, it takes a spirit of exploration to find more potential for progress.

As I said, a good routine is like the launchpad for a rocket. It gives you stability by working with your circumstances to stay consistent with your training. Your routine should also keep you pointing in the right direction by working your muscles in the right way.
Your job is to adapt and change your training routine however you see fit to fulfill those two objectives. Once you can do that, all you need to do is blast off to the heights you hope to reach by performing your exercises at a higher level over time.

I know it can be difficult to build a routine from scratch, so allow me to address some of the most common workout programming questions to bring more clarity to your planning. After that, I'll draw up some training templates to help get you started. After that, you can modify and change those templates to fit your needs.

Whole-body or split routine?

Adopting a split or full-body routine depends mostly on personal preference and lifestyle. Some people prefer to feel like they've worked the whole body and then enjoy several rest days. Others find they can focus on certain muscle groups more if they use a split routine.

I once noticed that I tended to slack off on my lower body exercises when doing full-body workouts. I would always start hitting my push and pull chain with a lot of energy but then call it a day after just one or two sets of squats. It was easier for me to work my legs with a split routine effectively. It allowed me to have a full workout dedicated to working just my squat and extension chains.

Split training can also emphasize each tension chain if you want to explore some second-level exercises regularly. Full body training typically prioritizes first-level exercises. The emphasis on compound exercises saves time as using many single and multi-joint exercises can bloat your workouts quickly. If you want to make the second-level exercises a primary staple, you may be better off with some split training.

Feel free to experiment with different plans and use the ones that seem to have the right combination that feels best for you. Some of the most common splits would be a push and pull split or an upper and lower body split.

PUSH/PULL 2-DAY SPLIT EXAMPLE

DAY 1 PUSH	DAY 2 PULL
ARCHER PUSH-UPS	PULL-UPS
SHOULDER PRESS	SINGLE -ARM ROWS
TRICEPS PRESS	BICEPS CURLS
HOVER LUNGES	SUSPENSION BRIDGE
SISSY SQUATS	HAMSTRING CURLS
STRETCH-OUTS	F.S. SIDE PLANK

UPPER/LOWER SPLIT WORKOUT EXAMPLE

DAY 1 UPPER
PULL-UPS
DIPS
REAR FLY
CHEST FLY
SIT-UPS

DAY 2 LOWER
PISTOL SQUATS
JUMP SQUATS
HIP EXTENSIONS
SIDE PLANKS

Chain training also makes it easy to split your workouts into movement chain and support chain workouts. The movement and support chain split is a favorite of many since the movement chains tend to be more taxing. In contrast, the support chains can be less metabolically demanding, so it feels like an active recovery day.

MOVEMENT/SUPPORT CHAIN SPLIT EXAMPLE

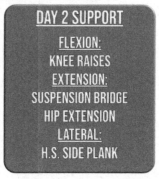

DAY 1 MOVEMENT
PUSH:
SINGLE-ARM PUSH-UP
OVERHEAD PRESS
PULL:
REAR FLY
SINGLE-ARM ROWS
SQUAT:
HOVER LUNGES

DAY 2 SUPPORT
FLEXION:
KNEE RAISES
EXTENSION:
SUSPENSION BRIDGE
HIP EXTENSION
LATERAL:
H.S. SIDE PLANK

Another fun tension chain split is to pair a movement chain with a support chain for three separate workouts. This approach gives you a balanced routine where you hit each tension chain twice a week and have one taxing movement chain with one slightly less taxing support chain.

MOVEMENT/SUPPORT CHAIN 3-DAY SPLIT EXAMPLE

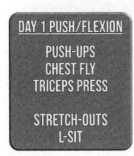
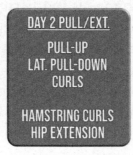
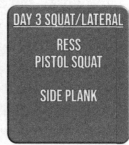

DAY 1 PUSH/FLEXION

PUSH-UPS
CHEST FLY
TRICEPS PRESS

STRETCH-OUTS
L-SIT

DAY 2 PULL/EXT.

PULL-UP
LAT. PULL-DOWN
CURLS

HAMSTRING CURLS
HIP EXTENSION

DAY 3 SQUAT/LATERAL

RESS
PISTOL SQUAT

SIDE PLANK

When should you make changes to your workout?

Like many aspects of diet and exercise, there's a balance between changing your routine while keeping things consistent and stable.

Changing your routine too often can compromise your training program's stability. Too much random change can leave you running around in circles without going anywhere. On the other hand, sticking to a strict workout that never changes can quickly become stale and limit the scope of your training.

One of the best solutions is to plan the changes in your routine every 4-6 weeks or so. Planning your changes gives you the stability of having a consistent routine and variation to change things. It also ensures that the changes aren't random and made without purpose. Planned changes tend to be more intentional and thought out, which helps ensure they are productive rather than detrimental.

Another option is to stick with your plan but make changes as needed. This ultra-flexible approach helps ensure you don't make unnecessary changes when they aren't warranted. At the same time, it gives you the freedom to go ahead and immediately switch things up without delay.

Sometimes change is warranted, but it's not always beneficial, so how can you know the change is in the right direction? The best way to know is to focus on what you're trying to train your muscles to do. Do you want your muscles to work harder so you get stronger? Are you trying to build stamina? Maybe you just want to perform better by increasing stability or power. You should clearly understand how a potential change can progress and how well you use your muscles. If the answer isn't clear, you risk adopting an unnecessary or detrimental change.

There's also always the very real possibility that a potential change won't make much difference. There are countless exercise and programing variations, but only a small percentage will make any meaningful difference. Most changes are just tweaks and adjustments that can change the flavor of the exercise but won't change how you're fundamentally using your muscles.

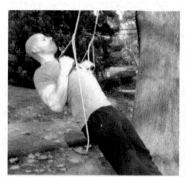 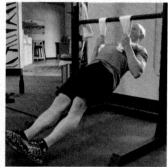

Changing tools and slight variations can make a common exercise feel fresh and new, but these changes may not make much difference if you still use your muscles the same way.

It's perfectly fine to change things up just for variety or if you like using a different exercise variation. If the change makes a big difference in what your muscles are doing, you're making some big changes to the stimulus you're creating. However, if you're still doing roughly the same amount of work with the muscles, you're still creating the same general stimulus.

How many times should you work each chain per week?

Training frequency depends on how much fatigue you induce due to both training volume and intensity. The harder you work your body, the longer you should recover before you train again.

Understanding the simple principle is crucial for breaking away from the dogmatic cookie-cutter training frequency recommendations you run across in our fitness culture. Some will claim you should only work a muscle once or twice weekly. Other coaches may recommend less frequency, like once a week or even every ten days. And yet, some coaches will claim training with a much higher frequency, in some cases working a muscle every day, is the way to go.

Both approaches are legitimate and can work very well. Remember, your training objective is not to work hard but to teach your muscles to work progressively harder over time. The *progression* of your routine gets results, not the actual routine itself.

Some people find they can progress if they work out more frequently, so they don't have to push themselves quite as hard in each workout. Others find it easier to progress if they train only once or twice a week and give themselves plenty of recovery.

Again, it boils down largely to personal preference. The important thing is to not be dogmatic in your training and make adjustments to give yourself the best chance to progress. If you are training three times a week, and find that the third workout is a struggle to get through, then you probably won't make much progress from that third workout. You'll probably be better off downshifting to twice a week. However, add an extra session per week if you feel you can handle it.

So those are some of the keys to getting what you want from your workout routine. I know it can be a little daunting to start from scratch, so here are some basic routine templates to help get you started. Feel free to change these up any way you like to suit your preferences and resources.

#10

DIY Suspension Rig

When I first got into suspension Calisthenics, I had difficulty finding equipment since it wasn't a very popular training method. Most big-name manufacturers were not producing quality straps at the time.

I started to experiment with building my suspension setups to save money and give myself more equipment options. Ironically, my interest in DIY suspension setups has been one of the most expensive aspects of my training career. I've built countless models and designs, and with every iteration, I would find flaws and things I liked.

Thankfully, more manufacturers have come to produce high-quality products like the ones from my favorite company, NOSSK. Since using their equipment, I haven't had much need to design my setup, especially since their quality and design are top-notch and their products are affordable.

DIY projects are still a lot of fun, and sometimes they can allow you to create equipment that may not be on the market. I've extensively covered most of my DIY setups in my second Book, Smart Bodyweight Training, but I wanted to share my latest design. It's a collection of highlights and benefits from all previous setups in one easy-to-use package.

Keep in mind that there is a certain level of risk and liability with all DIY fitness equipment. I feel very confident in the reliability of this design and the equipment I recommend; however, I know it has not been clinically tested, so please be cautious and use these at your own risk.

DIY suspension strap parts

This setup is super simple and ultra-minimalist. It uses only three pieces! The first is a single length of rope which you can find at your local outdoor retailer or online. I recommend the selection of 6 or 7mm ropes available through strapworks.com.

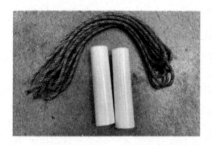 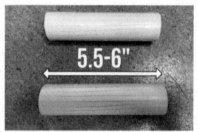

This rope should have minimal stretch and handle well over 1,000 pounds. I recommend selecting a length of around 14-16 feet, but feel free to select a length that suits your needs. Remember that you'll fold the rope in half, so purchase a rope at least twice the length for the height you want.

The other two pieces are the handles. I've always recommended cutting the handles from commercial cable machines in my past books. Those handles are purpose-built, comfortable, and well suited for suspension use. In the true spirit of DIY, some folks like to use PVC, which is cheaper and readily available in any hardware store.

PVC handles also allow you to cut them to the length you like, and you can make handles in various diameters to suit your hand size or grip preference. The downside to PVC is that cutting the plastic can lead to uneven and rough edges that pose a safety risk by wearing it on the ropes. I recommend the following steps to cut and finish your handles.

Step 1 Cut handles to length

I recommend using a tape measure to ensure both handles are the same length and cut each end using slow strokes of the saw to make the ends as square as possible. If you have access to a tool like a table, saw, or miter saw, that would be ideal for the perfect cut on both ends of the handles.

Step 2 Trim and sand down rough edges

Trim off any burrs and rough edges. I prefer to use a razor blade to do this. I also recommend shaving off the inside edge to create a smoother surface against the rope.

Once you've cut the burrs and rough edges, take a foam sanding block and sand down each end in a circular motion. This technique will give you a smooth surface on the end of the handle.

Step 3 Cut the grip texture

I used to wrap handles in hockey tape but found it can leave a sticky residue on my hands and get pretty dirty with use over time. Now, I just run the tip of a razor blade down the handle's length, creating a slightly raised line. Doing this around the whole handle will give you a reliable grip that's easy to clean and doesn't require extra parts or maintenance.

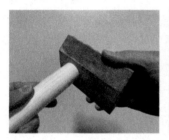 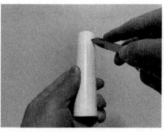 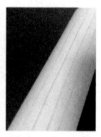

After cutting the handle to length, sand down any sharp and rough edges. Then score the grip texture with the tip of a razor blade.

You've now got your basic trainer once you have your rope and handles. All you need to do is to throw the rope over a sturdy support, like a thick tree limb, or you can feed the rope through a clinch knot on a pull-up bar.

Feed each end through the handle and attach the end with a bowline knot. Repeat on the other side. Refer to the tutorial at animatedknots.com to understand how to tie this knot.

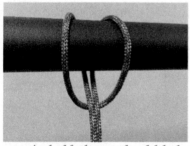 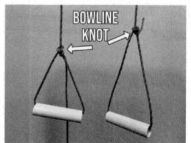

Fold the rope in half, throw the folded end over support and feed the rope back through. Tie each handle at the desired length with a bowline knot.

The bowline knot is a clinch knot, so the more weight you place on the handle, it will hold fast. It's also easy to undo by lifting on the loop, so you can easily change the height of your handles. You can also tie the loose end of the rope up, so it's out of the way if you wish.

This setup will accommodate almost any suspension exercise you need with a compact package to fit in your pocket. You can even feed the rope through the handle twice to create an adjustable self-locking foot sling.

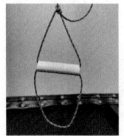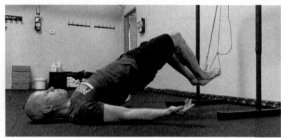

Feeding the rope through the handle a second time will give you an adjustable foot sling.

This design allows you to attach the trainer to almost any overhead anchor point, but there are a few adjustments you may want to make to suit the exercise you're planning to do. The first is to create a simple knotted loop, so the rope doesn't slip at the anchor point. This setup is useful for ensuring the rope doesn't slip if you place more weight on one handle during unilateral exercises.

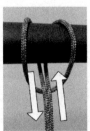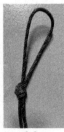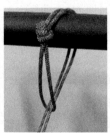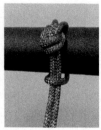

Creating a simple knotted loop can make the rope more secure so it doesn't slip when applying more weight onto one of the handles.

The second anchor adjustment is if you want to create a wider set of anchor points. This setup is more useful when performing pushing exercises like dips, push-ups, and chest flys. This anchor solution is commonly used with straight pull-up bars but can also work on tree branches. Just make sure you can reach up to the anchors to release them.

It can take some practice to set up this anchor point. You simply use the normal clinch knot on one side and then throw the rope over the bar and back under between the rope and the bar two more times at a wider point to create a second anchor.

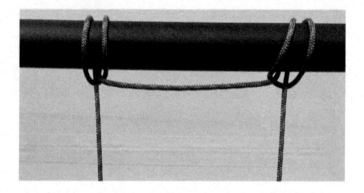

Additional DIY suspension accessories

The simple 3-piece DIY trainer is more than suitable on its own, but you can expand its versatility even further with a few basic accessories. Here are some of the more common ones I recommend.

Door anchor

The single length of rope will accommodate two out of the three potential suspension anchor points of overhead and out-of-reach anchors. If you want to use the trainer in a doorway, you'll need to fashion a door anchor to slip the rope through.

Thankfully this is an easy accessory to make; just fold a length of nylon and tie it in a knot. Cut the excess length off; voila, you have a handly door anchor. You can also use the knotted loop attachment mentioned earlier to create a more sturdy support for unilateral exercises.

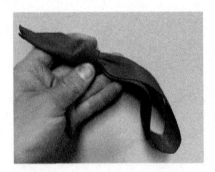 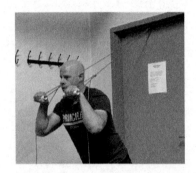

Foot loops

Building makeshift foot loops out of the rope is functionally sound, but it's not the most comfortable option, especially when training barefoot. Adding a simple pair of foot loops of nylon straps can go a long way toward a more comfortable experience.

There are two primary ways to add nylon foot loops to this trainer. The first is to buy a pair of simple cam buckle straps about one foot in length and half an inch wide.

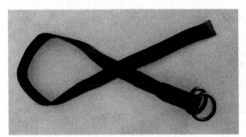 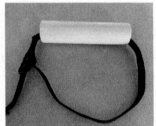

A simple 1.5' long nylon strap with a cam buckle or D-ring fastener can make a quick and handy adjustable foot loop easy to detach.

The simple solution is easy to install and remove. Plus, it allows some degree of adjustment for the size of your feet and footwear.

The second option is to invest in a pair of Simple Slings from strapworks.com. I recommend straps three feet in length and half an inch wide. The loops on each end should be about half an inch in diameter. This design requires more setup, but it gives you an adjustable foot loop that can instantly lockdown for a secure footing. The simple sling can also be a more comfortable strap that will lay flat against the forearm during push-ups and dips.

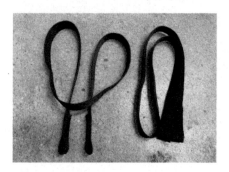 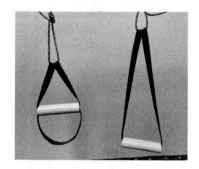

Pulley

One of the advantages of using a single piece of rope is you can run it through a pulley, which gives you some fun options for unique exercises.

The most common is pressing or pulling with only one arm while keeping the other arm tight to your side. This exercise is a relatively easy to start unilateral upper body training to work up to single-arm rows, pull-ups, and push-ups. The pulley also affords greater instability, making foot-suspended core exercises more challenging and dynamic.

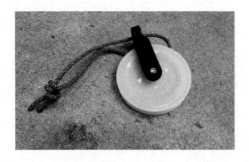 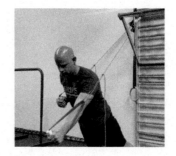

I recommend using a metal pulley over a plastic one you can find at your local hardware store. Simply attach it to an overhead support with a length of rope and feed the rope through the pulley before tying it on the other handle.

Towels and grip tools

The rope's simple nature means it can accommodate almost any attachment and accessory you might use on a cable machine. One of my favorites is using towels or specialized grip tools to give you different hand positions with basic exercises. You can adjust the standard handles to a vertical position, giving a similar experience. Still, specialized grip tools can make grip training and rotation more interesting.

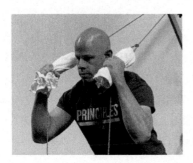 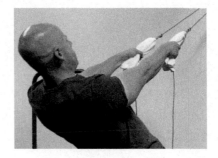

The important thing is to be creative but not get too carried away with crazy variations and exercise designs. The bulk of your progress will always come from the fundamental exercises discussed in this book, and this DIY trainer will certainly accommodate them. It's just nice to know that it will also be able to adapt to your changing circumstances.

#11

Trouble Shooting Suspension Workouts

Like all physical training methods, suspension calisthenics can be a very deep discipline that you can spend years exploring. This book is a starting point to give you some ideas and general guidelines. Feel free to further investigate this topic with the videos on my YouTube channel and podcast, and reach out to me (reddeltaproejct@gmail.com) with any questions. There's always more to learn. I've been obsessed over Suspension Calisthenics training for over a decade and feel like I'm barely scratching the surface.

Despite the simplicity of suspension calisthenics, it's only natural for challenges to crop up along your training journey. So allow me to take this opportunity to address some of the most common issues people have with their suspension work to give you the answers before they are needed, hopefully.

My arms keep rubbing the straps when doing push-ups and dips

Ideally, your arms will lightly touch the suspension straps while practicing pushing chain movements, but there shouldn't be any harsh abrasion.

There are several things you can do to remedy this. The first is to have a wider anchor point if possible. When you have a narrow or single anchor point, the straps form an inverted V, leaving less room for your body to pass through.

Another solution is to keep the arms as tight to the side of the body as possible. This technique prevents rubbing against the straps and reduces the stress on the shoulders.

It's common for people to spread their arms out to the side even though they feel as tight to the torso as possible. Taking a video of yourself doing push-ups and dips can be a humbling yet enlightening experience. There's often a difference between how we think we're moving and performing.

Lastly, keeping the arms into the sides is more challenging if you have trouble retracting and depressing your shoulder blades, especially as you descend into the bottom of a push-up position. Your arms will naturally be forced outward and pressed against the straps if your shoulders hunch up.

Packing the shoulders down and back as much as possible helps make your torso more narrow and allows your arms to tuck into your sides. Packing the shoulders will also offer more stability for your shoulders and reduce joint stress.

What if I have joint pain?

Joint pain is the most common chronic injury associated with physical activity. Suspension calisthenics is typically pretty joint-friendly, but it's impossible to eliminate any risk of joint injury in any training method. Some of the most common sites for joint pain are the knees, shoulders, lower back, and elbows.

Unfortunately, there can be any number of causes of joint pain and discomfort, ranging from structural injury, like arthritis or a torn ligament, to a lack of proper limb alignment.

Furthermore, joint discomfort may have little to do with the area where you feel the strain. Lower back pain is often the result of weak hamstrings or a slouching posture. Shoulder discomfort can originate from improper neck alignment or back strength.

The plethora of possible causes is why I advise seeing a health professional diagnose the issue firsthand. Trying to assess and self-diagnose joint issues over the Internet can quickly have you running around in circles. One-on-one guidance can give you more clarity on what's causing the issue to fix the problem quickly.

In the meantime, avoid any exercises or movements that aggravate the condition and train around the injury. It's also a good idea to take care of the issue quickly. Joint pain and discomfort will always hold you back, and there is no way to work around injury without losing some progress. So don't go several months or even years "dealing" with the issue. Get it fixed asap.

What do I do if I can't find a place to hang my straps?

Finding a place to hang your straps is usually not a problem in your daily environment. Most people will find or build a reliable place to hang their straps in the home or outside. Here are a few tips if you're having issues finding a place to hang your straps while on the road or looking for new places to train.

Use the Maps application on your smartphone to find parks and recreation areas. These spaces often have monkey bars and sometimes even dedicated pull-up stations where you can hang your straps. If nothing else, parks generally have manicured trees that offer suitable branches for hanging your straps.

Keep an eye out for stairways and high railings. These areas are especially handy when staying in a hotel and you don't have or want to use a door anchor in your hotel room. Stairways are usually constructed with sturdy metal and can be a suitable place to hang your trainer from an overhead landing.

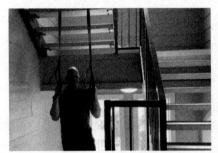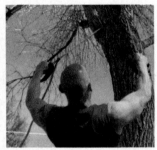

Stairways and tree limbs offer the perfect place to use your suspension straps. Just use caution around such inconsistent environments.

Just be mindful of the structural integrity of whatever you're hanging your straps from and the flooring surface underneath it. If you are hanging in the stairway, you may be stepping down onto a set of stairs that can be less safe to land on. Always be aware of rough surfaces or sharp edges that can compromise the integrity of the anchor point. It doesn't take much to tear or break a strap when under tension during an exercise.

Finding places to use your straps can seem problematic when you are new to suspension calisthenics, but you will quickly develop an eye for good places to get your work out. It won't be long before you instinctively notice ideal places to hang your straps in almost any environment.

Should I pair my training with any special diet?

Diet and exercise seem to go together like water and sand at the beach. Sound nutrition is also important when weight management is one of your fitness goals. The fitness media is also saturated with messages telling you that you should be ingesting all sorts of supplements and using a special diet. Such messages have conditioned us to believe we need a special diet to go along with our workout program.

Most folks do not practice enough intense or long-duration exercise to require any special nutritional changes aside from what constitutes a normal healthy diet. Influences like your height, body type, weight management goals, genetics, and other lifestyle factors are more important to your dietary needs than what you may do in a typical workout.

That's not to say that diet isn't extremely important; it certainly is. It's just not always important whether or not you're exercising. I'm sure you probably don't need me to show you the basics of sound nutrition, but there's a lot of confusion with conflicting messages on what constitutes a healthy diet.

Here at the Red Delta project, a healthy diet is one that adequately satisfies your four primal appetites. These include your hunger, nutritional support, metabolic and energy support, and the enjoyment you gain from food. Except for medical conditions, like food sensitivities and allergies, there is no standard dietary rule or practice that you have to follow.

So stick to the basics, eat enough to satisfy your hunger, and get plenty of nutrient-dense foods for nutritional support. Pay attention to how your diet influences your energy level and ability to feel good throughout the day and during your workout. Above all else, eat foods that you enjoy and treat yourself occasionally. A diet that leaves you feeling deprived and fighting chronic cravings can hardly be considered healthy.

There is a chance that ramping up your physical activity may increase your hunger, especially if you've been fairly sedentary. An increase in hunger is not bad and is by no means something to worry over. Simply add a bit of extra protein-rich or nutrient-dense foods to cover that increased calorie demand. You probably won't need to ingest any special supplement or a lot of extra food. An extra couple of eggs at breakfast or a handful of trail mix as a snack in the afternoon will probably cover you just fine.

I keep feeling conflicted over what to do. How do you address workout FOMO?

There's always someone coming out with a new revolutionary, life-changing program or exercise method. It's only natural to feel like you would be missing out on this incredible opportunity if you didn't adopt it immediately.

If you're not missing out on the latest trends, you may fall into constant fear-mongering rabbit holes. Some experts preach how any approach other than their own will spell disaster.

These messages can become emotionally taxing and distract you from putting your efforts into what matters most; your actual training. The irony is that chasing after every new trend can compromise the stability of your training routine, thus jeopardizing your ability to make progress. The more you chase different rabbits, the lesser your chance of catching one.

Identifying the fundamental principles of fitness and exercise helps you cut through that noise. All past, present, and future training methods are potentially effective for the same fundamental reasons. Anything that will help you get stronger will do so because it will challenge your strength. Any effective weight loss strategy will have you consume fewer calories or burn more energy.

So go ahead and change your diet and workout program any way you like, especially if you desire to make such changes. Don't worry about whatever new methods someone else is excited or worried over. If you don't feel it's in alignment with your preferences, resources, and lifestyle, it's probably not helpful.

I keep having doubts about my ability to reach my goals. What can I do to restore faith in myself?

It's natural to experience periods of doubt and question what you're doing in your ability to achieve results. After all, you're trying to do something you've never done before, so uncertainty will be part of the game as you explore your potential.

Periods of doubt can be more prevalent when you experience setbacks or make mistakes. Once again, this is natural and happens to anyone who dares to journey off the beaten path. Understanding doubt and mistakes are part of growth and can signify that you're on the right track.

The first thing to do during self-doubt is to continue taking action. It doesn't matter if you're doing something as big as running five miles a day or simply having a healthy breakfast each morning; productive action is the best way to reduce self-doubt. "Taking a break" and no longer putting one foot in front of the other will only serve to reinforce your doubts.

It can also be helpful to seek out the guidance of a coach. I'm not referring to electronic aids like a smartphone app or a YouTube video. Sitting down and talking about your concerns with another human being in person or over video chat can help you address your fears and overcome personal obstacles.

Lastly, invite some flexibility into your training program. Keeping a strict and rigid routine can inhibit the opportunities to grow and keep moving forward. Self-doubt usually creeps in when you find yourself doing the same old thing repeatedly as a matter of routine. Adopting a more playful approach, where you can change your training, can do wonders.

Can suspension calisthenics help with fat loss?

There's no such thing as an effective fat loss exercise. It's all about progressing the *functional* demands upon your body. You can train to be stronger, faster, mobile, stable, and more stamina. However, it's not possible to train skinny.

Don't feel discouraged, though, because any physical movement can influence fat loss and weight management. A calorie burned is a calorie burned regardless of why it's used in the first place. Burning 100 calories will have the same influence whether you're walking the dog, running up a mountain, or doing push-ups.

That's not to say that some exercise methods may not make it easier to burn more calories than others. Time is one of the most significant variables in helping you burn energy. The longer you're physically active, the more fat and calories you burn. Naturally, activities you spend a longer period doing will burn significantly more calories.

On the surface, it may seem like suspension calisthenics can't burn many calories, especially since you can get a decent workout in less than half an hour. This assumption is correct, but many secondary influences toward fat loss come with suspension calisthenics.

For one, building muscle and strength benefits your ability to burn energy. Muscle is like the engine of the human body, and bigger engines typically burn more energy when put to use. Not only that, but stronger muscles can also work at a higher level of intensity for longer periods. You can think about strength training as an effective way to upgrade your body's potential to burn more energy. The stronger and more resilient you make your body, the easier it will be to burn more fat.

Strength training can also improve mobility and joint health. Few things are more fattening than pain. Building a body that feels good in motion will make it easier to be active for longer periods and at higher intensities.

I've been training for a while now, but the gains are not coming as I hoped. What am I doing wrong?

Technically, there's no such thing as a fruitless exercise or workout. Everything you do in your training works 100% effectiveness 100% of the time. Your body will always adapt to the functional demands you place upon it. When you feel like a workout isn't working, it's usually due to a misalignment between your expectations and what you're telling your body. Therefore, getting a workout to "work" is just a matter of adjusting your approach to align expectations and demand. Here are several reasons why such misalignment may be occurring.

Not enough intensity

Lack of intensity is a very common issue in bodyweight-based exercise discipline. Lack of training intensity is also why many claim that you can't build muscle and strength with bodyweight training. To be fair, it can be very difficult to effectively build up your body when you lack intensity in your training. That's why it's important to understand the basic progressive concepts discussed in this book to push your muscles with a high resistance level.

Suspension Calisthenics can make it easier to explore high levels of intensity. You can find yourself in trouble if you try to lift too much weight in the gym. However, If you put too much weight on your hands during a push-up, you can just step forward and reduce the intensity.

So if you feel things are not progressing the way you want, go ahead and load up your hands or feet and see how hard you can push the resistance.

Failure to take other influences into account

All success comes from several variables, and focusing too much on one or two (how many reps you can do, how much protein you eat, and so on) can distract you from other influences that may be holding you back.

It's hard to say what other variables you should focus on as there are countless directions you can focus your attention. A good rule of thumb, though, is what's holding you back are the things you know you need to focus on in the back of your mind.

The cardio junkie who can't seek to lose weight may never miss a workout, but they turn a blind eye to the half a dozen sodas they drink every day. The hard-core lifter isn't building muscle because they are afraid to eat more, so they continue to eat like a bird in fear of getting fatter. The health nut with the perfect diet and workout program knows their late-night Netflix binges continue to leave them tired and prone to getting sick. When you're struggling to progress, chances are pretty good you won't move the needle by trying to optimize the areas you already focus on. It's more often the influences you're continuing to ignore.

Trying to out-work a lack of progression or proficiency

It's always tempting to double down on your efforts and vow to work harder when not getting what you want from your training. Sometimes working harder can help, but this is usually a temporary solution since you can't scale hard work indefinitely.

"Working harder" can also often mean doing more than you already do. You do more cardio, sets, and workouts and add more restrictions to your diet. Doing more of the same can sometimes help, but it usually creates a lot of redundancy that costs you much more time and energy. You essentially spend more resources just to reinforce what you've already got.

There are a couple of cases when doing more can help. The first is if your training has been inconsistent or follows a start-stop-start pattern. On-and-off habits can certainly undermine your progress, so I first try to identify inconsistencies when clients struggle.

The second time doing more can help if you're not exercising very much in the first place. If you're only working out once a week or doing an exercise you are struggling with once in a while, then yes, doing it more may help.

But let's say you're already consistently putting in a solid effort. In that case, squeezing out a bit more work is more likely to burn you out with little more to show for it. It's vital to gain insight into what things you can do differently instead of doing the same things more. This instance is where having an outside opinion from a coach or mentor can help. Getting a second pair of eyes on your situation can be invaluable in identifying weaknesses or mistakes you didn't know you were making.

How can I combine suspension calisthenics with other types of strength training?

I've never believed in following any single approach or method for either diet or exercise. All methods have their pros and cons. Combining multiple modalities keeps you interested and fills in the gaps that leave you vulnerable to injury and burnout. Feel free to combine suspension calisthenics with powerlifting, yoga, or anything else that suits you and your goals.

The biggest risk with combining modalities is that adding too many exercises can quickly bloat your workouts, leaving you to spend far more time and effort than necessary. Most training bloat comes from redundancy, where you create the same stimulus using different methods. You're using various tools and techniques, but fundamentally, you're just using your muscles the same way repeatedly.

The best way to reduce redundancy is to program around a tension chain approach. So instead of thinking of different exercises or methods, you return to the fundamental perspective of push chain movements or squat chain movements. This perspective keeps things categorized into the same general stimuli for various methods.

SQUAT CHAIN EXERCISES:	PUSH CHAIN EXERCISES:
- LEG PRESS	- BENCH PRESS
- HACK SQUAT	- PUSH-UPS
- LUNGES	- DIPS
- LEG EXTENSIONS	- CABLE CHEST FLY
- PISTOL SQUATS	- CABLE PRESS DOWN
- JUMPING	- HANDSTAND
- SPRINTING	- LAT. D.B. RAISE

There are many great ways to work every tension chain, but you only need a few basic exercises that are right for you.

Chain training gives you the freedom and flexibility to swap out methods for your exercises. For example, a barbell bench press, suspension archer push-up, and weight machine chest press are all push chain exercises. They even use the same basic movement pattern. So even though they may be different exercises in a workout log, they'll create the same general stimulus.

I recommend just mixing and swapping out the exercises as you wish. You may do suspension archer push-ups for your push chain exercise in one workout. Then, in the next push chain workout, you use the weight machine chest press. This way, you're changing up what you're doing as far as your method, but fundamentally you're still creating the same progressive stimulus and staying on track with your workout program.

An exercise is supposed to work muscle X, but I feel it in muscle Y; what am I doing wrong?

You may not be doing anything wrong, which may even be good. It's not uncommon for people to feel a weaker muscle along a tension chain working harder. Common examples may include feeling your triceps working during push-ups or your hip flexors working while doing sit-ups.

Most of the time, this is just exposing a weak muscle along the chain, which will resolve as you continue to practice the exercise. That muscle will become stronger, and even though it's still working as part of that chain, it's no longer the weak link that feels like it's working harder.

Other times, you may not feel a target muscle working because you have difficulty contracting it in the first place. This scenario is not uncommon and is one of the primary reasons people have lagging muscle groups.

The solution for this issue is to practice a few simple isometric exercises that target the muscle group beforehand. Doing so will improve your ability to engage and warm up your neuromuscular connection. This practice should improve your ability to contract the muscle on command and feel it working harder during the basic exercise. You can learn more about overcoming isometric exercises on the isometrics playlist on the Red Delta Project YouTube channel and in my book, *Overcoming Isometrics*.

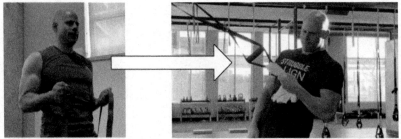

I'm doing an isometric curl with an isoloop strap to engage my biceps and help them work better during my single-arm suspension towel rows.

How many exercises should I use in a workout?

Beware of the temptation always to add more exercises to a workout routine. The more techniques you have, the more time and energy the workout will cost you. There's also the tendency to dilute the intensity of your workout across many exercises. Furthermore, many potential exercises are just slight variations of the ones you're already doing. You may be spending a lot of time just practicing redundant movements that don't bring any additional benefit beyond what you gained with the first exercise.

In most cases, one to two basic compound movements is usually sufficient to create a powerful stimulus. There's usually very little need for half a dozen exercises, especially when they all fundamentally do the same thing.

My general rule of thumb is to make sure that each exercise in a workout creates a very different stimulus from before. There are several ways to do this, and I encourage you to apply these elements as much as possible.

Change from bilateral to unilateral movements

Suspension Calisthenics makes it easy to switch from using both limbs simultaneously to doing exercises that use one arm or leg independent of the other. Switching from a bilateral to a unilateral technique can bring in a lot of new challenges.

Common examples may include single-arm pushing and pulling or squatting movements to lunging movements.

Change speed and tempo

Exercise speed is a fun thing to play around with, and most people get stuck with a moderate repetition tempo. Try doing an exercise at your normal speed and then do the next set faster or slower than before.

Some fun examples may include going from slow squats to jumping or fast tempo push-ups to slow push-ups.

Change resistance

Like repetition speed, most people get stuck working with the same resistance level and use the same repetition range with all their exercises.

There's nothing wrong with having a standard level of resistance you feel is best for you. However, it's good to change the resistance periodically so you expose your muscles to a broader variety of stimuli. It's also very effective to keep your mind engaged and maintaining interest in your workouts.

Change your angle to gravity

This one applies a little more to the upper body, where you may do a vertical pushing or pulling movement instead of a horizontal pushing or pulling movement. So in one exercise, you may do push-ups, and in the next, you could be doing pike push-ups. Going from pull-ups into rows is another common example.

The key here is to ensure that every exercise in your training arsenal brings unique benefits and stimuli. Suppose you're going to put the time and effort into doing an additional exercise; you want to get as much benefit as possible. It's much better to do that than to do five different push-up variations that essentially do the same thing.

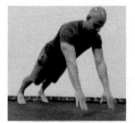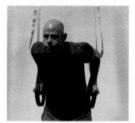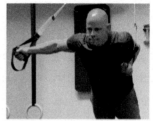

Each of these push chain exercises brings something unique to the workout.

How should I use suspension calisthenics for cardio?

I primarily use suspension calisthenics for developing strength and building muscle. That's not to say it can't be a useful tool for jacking up the heart rate and developing some cardiovascular conditioning.

Here are some of the most effective ways to practice suspension calisthenics with a cardio element.

Circuit training

One of the easiest ways to create a higher metabolic demand is to do the same strength workout you normally do, with less rest between sets and exercises.

Technically the line between strength training and cardio exists only in our imagination. All types of physical activity require some strength, just as all movement creates a metabolic demand. Even standing up from a chair requires strength in your legs and increased metabolic response.

We typically consider cardiovascular exercise as just an activity that requires a lot of metabolic activity relative to rest. Therefore, decrease the amount of rest, and you can achieve a cardiovascular benefit from your strength training.

Integrate cardio burst activity

Cardioburst exercises are techniques that can quickly create a high metabolic demand and typically last only a few minutes. Common examples are skipping rope, sprinting, plyometrics like box jumps, or doing a few hundred meters on a rowing machine.

Integrating cardio burst exercises with your suspension calisthenics can do wonders for jacking your heart rate without costing you a lot of additional time and energy. It can also be more enjoyable since you don't have to spend countless soul-sucking minutes watching the clock tick down on a treadmill.

I recommend doing these cardio burst activities after a suspension exercise, especially if building muscle and strength is your primary goal. It's much more difficult to create a stimulus for building yourself up when you are winded and out of breath.

Do cardio with suspension exercises

The portability of suspension equipment opens the door for a fun training possibility that you otherwise may not have with heavier weight-based equipment.

You can enjoy your traditional outdoor cardio exercise while carrying a suspension strap. You set up your strengths and get a quick strength session before continuing your run.

I've done this several times while going out for a hike and finding a suitable tree to do some pull-ups and dips. If you live near a park or recreation area, you can jog or ride a bike there, set up for a workout, and then jog or ride home.

This training can be fun to break up the monotony of a longer cardio session while enjoying the outdoors and getting much-needed vitamin D in the sunshine.

Conclusion

Well, my friend, you've reached the end of the book and potentially the beginning of your suspension calisthenics training career. Usually, books like this end with a message of hope about how what you've learned can potentially change your body and your life. But I'm not going to take that route.

Instead, I believe it's much more important to remember that, like all strength training methods, suspension calisthenics isn't anything special, unique, or different. It works for the same reason all strength training methods work; by bringing progressive resistance against your major muscle groups through fundamental movement patterns.

The truly special elements are the discipline, focus, skill, and intensity you bring to your training to make it effective. There is no magic workout formula or special ingredient to achieving the desired results. Those looking for such things end up running around in circles on a wild goose chase hopping from one program to the next.

I hope that suspension Calisthenics can bring you some of the solutions you've been looking for and enhance your training, but remember that what you bring to your workouts is far more important than what the workouts bring you.

So I bid you ado and leave you on your journey, But remember that you don't have to go it alone. I'm always available through my Red Delta Project and email at reddeltaproject@gmail.com to answer any questions you have along your journey.

Be fit, live free,

Matt Schifferle

About the Author

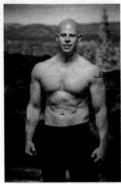

- Matt Schifferle is the founder of the Red Delta Project, an online resource dedicated to helping you maximize your results through minimalist fitness strategies.

- You can learn more at https://www.reddeltaproject.com and discover more on the Red Delta Project YouTube channel. You can also search for the Red Delta Project Podcast in your favorite podcast directory.

- Feel free to reach out to Matt through email (**reddeltaproject@gmail.com**) or you can DM him on Instagram @red.delta.project.

- Look for these other R.D.P titles, in paperback and Kindle format on Amazon:

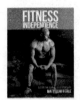 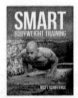 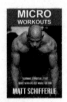

Printed in Great Britain
by Amazon

26675485R10097